MW00961664

Intermittent Fasting:

Everything You Need to Know About Intermittent Fasting for Beginner to Expert — Build Lean Muscle and Change Your Life

James Sinclair

James-Sinclair

© Copyright 2016- All rights reserved

without the consent of the author or copyright owner. Legal action will be pursued if this is breached.

Table of Contents

James-Sinclair

Introduction

When was the last time you ate? An hour ago? Several hours? Yesterday? Are you starving, feeling like you are going to die of starvation? That's how most of us feel at one time or another. We ate breakfast a few hours ago and then we get that hungry feeling in our stomachs.

Intermittent fasting will teach you how to read your body in terms of hunger pangs. It will teach you that hunger has a peak point, after which it quickly disappears. After a little while, even if you haven't eaten for several hours, you really don't feel that hungry.

Intermittent fasting—sounds interesting, doesn't it? It's not exactly a diet, per se; it cuts down on what you eat, yet also ensures that you get your fill of calories through wholesome foods. Picture this — you skip breakfast each day, eat two meals at spaced intervals later on, say, at around 1 pm and 8 pm. Then nothing at all till the next morning. Did you just shrink back in horror? How is this possible? How can I live for so long without eating? What about my metabolism? My workout routine will also go for a toss. How will I build muscle mass?

Relax. You won't keel over and pass out by the end of the first day of intermittent fasting. People who have practiced it report increased muscle mass, decreased body fat, increased explosiveness while lifting weights, drastic reduction in their training time, and generally being at the top of their game, all the while eating less and continuing their exercise schedules and work routines. Sounds like a recipe for increased muscle building efficiency and optimal weight loss. It's been shown to be possible while maintaining a healthy, albeit reduced dietary plan, even when that plans involves fasting.

In fact, those hunger pangs won't return until about 20-24 hours later, but they will never be as bad as they were the first time. There is a good reason for this wave of hunger, a scientific one. It all comes down to hormones — insulin, norepinephrine, epinephrine, leptin, glucagon and ghrelin — and the response your organs make to these hormones.

For those of you that are conscious of your fitness and are used to eating three meals a day or grazing on five or six smaller ones, the thought of fasting or going without food is probably putting fear into you right now. Most people who are active start to get hungry around four or five hours after a meal and some go to the extremes of panicking, the alarm bells start ringing and your body starts screaming at you, "Feed me! If you don't feed me you're gonna die of starvation, you're gonna lose all that muscle you've built up!" We are so frequently told that our bodies need to eat, and eat often, in order to gain lean, strong muscle mass that we rarely even consider alternatives for fear of losing what we have worked so hard to gain but evidence suggests that the option of eating less often might be well worth investigating.

In fact, as you will see as you read this book, that won't happen. What will more than likely happen is that you will shed a bit of that excess body fat. Research has shown that intermittent fasting can help to get the fat burning process in your body revved up as well as helping to control the levels of glucose and insulin in your body. The control of the hormones in your body and the corresponding changes could result in a decrease in your body fat and increase in your muscle mass, just by skipping out on a meal or two. This method can enable you to reach your fitness goals and shed the stubborn fat layers that remain, just by branching out into territory that many fitness aficionados have never dared to explore, to their own peril.

What you will most definitely lose, and I promise that you will feel totally liberated by this, is that unfounded fear that if you don't eat every few hours, you will waste away. And, you can still eat every few hours, depending on which intermittent fast plan you choose. Like most good diets, intermittent fasting offers flexibility, enabling you to custom tailor your own unique dietary plan in order to ensure fantastic results targeting your own personal goals. It's not as simple as just not eating anymore. The results, by way of fat loss and muscle gain, will speak for themselves. Plus, at the end of the day, you will have gained something even more important — perspective. You will learn to see food differently and you will learn to listen to your body. Discovering for yourself what your body needs to stay energized and healthy will grant you a whole different viewpoint on yourself and on the food you consume every day, and, in doing so, will enable you to reach a whole new level of fitness.

If you are ready to start, step into the world of intermittent fasting and be prepared for your life to be shaken up and turned upside down — all in a good way!

James-Sinclair

Chapter 1

What Is Fasting?

Fasting is the voluntary act of avoiding food, either partially or completely, for a pre-determined amount of time, often for religious purposes. In particular, Christianity and Islam are two of the most ardent proponents of fasting as their members believe that by depriving the body of food for some fixed period of time; they feed their spirits, atone for their sins, gain the favor of God or atone for their sins. Muslims practice fasting more, most notably during the celebration of Ramadan. Many Christians also fast not as a requirement but as a choice, the examples being set by Jesus Christ and many biblical personalities. Such fasting can range from simply not consuming certain food objects (such as the common abstaining from meat demonstrated by Catholics observing Lent) to complete restraint from consuming any food or beverages outside of water at all (usually done by the devout as a deeply personal choice).

Spiritual Strength

It is believed that fasting makes one stronger in the spirit. The primary basis for this is the principle of the flesh vs. the spirit, i.e., the more you indulge the flesh, the weaker your spirit becomes. It's this tug-of-war between the two that gives fasting its spiritual importance.

From a secular perspective, particularly a psychological one, this belief is still valid to a great extent. Why? The principle of delayed gratification. Fasting is one of the best ways to exercise delayed gratification and instill self-discipline. A strong spirit is generally a strong mind and by fasting, you train your mind to hold off on that, which is very, very hard to resist: a deliciously legitimate need called food. And since the mind is like a muscle, fasting on a regular basis is very good mental exercise. Exercising your mind is as important as exercising your body, and will instill in you the discipline and self-control needed to reach your personal fitness goals. Plus, that food tastes so much better after you've waited for it.

Benefits of Fasting

You may ask how is purposefully allowing yourself to be hungry for extended periods of time beneficial to your health and well-being? Isn't it bad to let yourself be hungry for long periods of time? I mean that's why we have to eat, right?

I know what you mean. At first glance, going hungry doesn't seem like a good idea for better health. However, the truth is, fasting — if done right — can actually be very good for all aspects of your health, including physical, psychological, and emotional health.

According to the Swiss-German Renaissance man Paracelsus, fasting is the greatest cure and our internal doctor, and many people agree with him. Fasting has been referred to as the body's "miracle cure" due to the many physical conditions or ailments that many people report to have been alleviated by fasting. The most common conditions that can reportedly be alleviated by fasting include:

· Allergies;

· Arthritis;

· Asthma;

· Cardiovascular Ailments;

· Digestive Problems; and

· Skin Diseases.

How is this so? One reason is fasting's reported ability to initiate, kick-start, or reset the body's natural healing mechanism.

Another reported benefit of fasting is, surprisingly, increased energy. And it does so first by helping us curb our tendencies to go overboard with food, i.e., regular binging. Food is great, no doubt about it. Yet, excess amounts of even the best things in life can be detrimental in the long run. In the case of food, regularly overeating increases our bodies' burdens. Think back on times when you've indulged in a bit too much food. How active did you feel after? Likely you were not at your most energetic—sluggish, slightly nauseous, and bloated.

Consider how you felt after you were given an abnormally

Fasting is the time you give your body the opportunity to take a break from the deluge of food and the workload associated with having to properly digest and process the food. Eating does give us energy but digesting food also requires energy. The process of digestion, assimilation and metabolism of food needs significant amounts of energy and experts estimate that 65% of the body's energy goes to digesting food after each heavy meal. Cutting out a sizable amount of that energy demand enables your body to better focus the time it would have used digesting those unnecessary meals into processes essential for your health. These processes are directly undermined when you eat too often.

Breaking a long or short fast

You need to break your fast properly to avoid any undesirable consequences. Gobbling up too much food after breaking your fast can result in a critical condition known as the re-feeding syndrome. When you introduce too much food into your body after fasting for a while, there's a rapid shift from ketosis to carbohydrate-based food, which prompts the body to supply an excess amount of insulin to quickly digest all the carbs. This process needs large amounts of magnesium, potassium, phosphates and vitamins such as Vitamin B1 (Thiamine), which are usually severely depleted when you've been fasting for any amount of time. This sudden need for large quantities of these nutrients leads to severe deficiencies, resulting in heart failure, hypotension, and possibly sudden death.

Some helpful guidelines for avoiding this syndrome include:

Don't rush: Ensure that you start slow. You can begin with an intake of 10 calories/kg of body weight daily or 5 calories/kg if you fasted for longer than fifteen days. Then make a daily increase of 5 calories/kg.

Use liquids: Break your fast with diluted fruit juice or bone broth, which are both loaded with electrolytes. If possible, squeeze the juice yourself but if you have to buy it, make sure that it is pure juice devoid of sugar and other additives.

Bit by bit: Longer fasts will require a longer time to break.

If you fast for longer than a week, you'll need to gradually and carefully reintroduce solid foods to your body. Do not do it all at once.

Eat slowly: Eat small portions slowly. After a while, as your body starts to adjust to having food again, transition to foods such as cream of tomato soup or sweet potato lime soup, which are perfect for consumption. Also, well-cooked vegetables, egg yolks, and a bone broth soup are rich sources of healthy fats, protein, and nutrients.

Use supplements if required: About thirty minutes before breaking your fast, supplement with thiamine and other B vitamins, sodium, magnesium, potassium and phosphorus. This will help your body begin to digest the food you are about to consume.

Kinds of Fasts

Generally speaking, there are 2 general ways to fast: total and partial. A total fast is one where you avoid food in all its forms and drink only water during the fasting period, which is at least 24 hours. As the name denotes, partial fasts are those during which you don't completely give up food — you can choose to just give up a particular food item or items, or limit your complete fast to just a few hours, or both.

Categories of Fasting Methods

As explained before, fasting can be done for various reasons including detox, cleansing, religious purposes, treating a health condition, and weight loss. Your preferred fasting method should be suitable for your body's chemistry and overall health needs and desires. If you're on medication or have a sensitive medical condition but you desire to partake in a fast, ensure that you speak with your healthcare provider before taking the next step.

With that aside, these are the categories of fasting and their associated methods:

Dry Fasting

Dry fasting is also commonly referred to as Hebrew Fast, Black Fast or Absolute Fast and it is the most extreme category of fasting. With spiritual origins, this type of fasting involves giving up food and water for short periods. **Religious fasts** fall under this category. People enter into religious fasts for primarily spiritual reasons. A good example of such fast is the Daniel Fast, which is fashioned after the Biblical book of Daniel. This fast prohibits every kind of food except grains, vegetables, fruits and water for about 21 days. Some other types of religious fasts are the Jewish Tzomot (involves a group of fasts spread out within an entire year) and the Ramadan (a one-month fast where Muslims refrain from food from sunrise until sundown).

Liquid fasting

As the name implies, only liquids are taken during this fast. Depending on the liquid used during the fast, there are different kinds of liquid fasts. A **Juice Fast** is probably the most favorite type of liquid fast, as it provides a modicum of nutritional sustenance in a natural and pure form. Juice fasting entails consuming only the liquids from vegetables and fruits and forbids the intake of solid food for a specific period, which can run from one day to two weeks. Although you may need to do some planning to certify that you get sufficient minerals and vitamins, juice fasting is quite simple, as fruits and vegetables can be obtained with ease. A food processor, blender or juicer can be used to process these fruits and veggies, and the pulp can be mixed with water, and consumed about five times daily.

Water fasting is the oldest and simplest type of liquid

fasting. With it, you can derive immense therapeutic and physical benefits in a short time because detox happens more rapidly. However, water fasting is quite stringent and may be really challenging for a beginner. Also, it should not be carried out without checking with your doctor. Depending on your goals and physical conditions, about 2 qt. of pure water should be consumed every day. Water fasts that are medically monitored had remarkable effects on stabilizing blood pressure.

A cleansing fast, also known as the Lemonade Diet or Master Cleanse, is a fairly recent approach and involves a liquid drink containing lemon juice, pure maple syrup (for calories) and a spice, such as cayenne pepper. The principal purpose of this fast is intestinal cleansing which rids the colon of toxins and foods. For maximum effect, this liquid is to be taken 6 to 12 times every day. A laxative tea, which is a more concentrated form of cleansing, can be taken two times every day, in the morning and evening. A typical cleansing fast may last for up to two weeks. However, for longer fasts, there must be professional supervision to prevent adverse consequences.

The Liquid Protein Fast is mainly used by obese

patients for weight loss. A liquid protein fast can be hugely beneficial to those who need to lose weight ranging from 10 to 100lbs. Like the water fast, medical supervision is required to ensure that all the nutrients and minerals you need are provided.

A **Diagnostic Fast** can be implemented for various testing purposes. They usually involve a complete abstinence from food or liquids except water for about 8 to 12 hours before testing. For example, a fasting glucose tolerance test used to measure glucose levels in the blood requires a diagnostic fast. You may also be placed on a diagnostic fast for certain surgical procedures.

Partial Fasting

Partial fasting is usually known as selective fasting and will include or exclude certain kinds of solid foods, such as meats, rice, and wheat. Some partial fasts restrict the amount of food consumed to less than three whole meals, while other partial fasts can limit certain kind of foods in your meal. Some examples are mono diets, such as rice fasting, and cleansing diets.

Some Other Types of Fasting Methods

<u>Daily Intermittent Fasting</u>

This is modeled on the Leangains model, which uses a 16 hour fast, followed by an 8 hour eating period. It doesn't matter when you begin your eating period. It's completely your wish — you may start at 8 am and end at 4 pm, or begin at 2 pm and end at 10 pm. Do what works best for you. Because this kind of fasting is done every day, it is easy to get into a habit of eating according to this schedule. If you are accustomed to eating at certain times in a day, all you have to change is the time — you just learn not to eat at certain times, which becomes easier with time.

The potential limitation of this method is that you might not ingest the requisite number of calories per day, as you will cut out one or two meals from your plan. It might get difficult for you to make yourself eat bigger meals in a limited time frame, resulting in losing weight unnecessarily.

<u>Weekly Intermittent Fasting</u>

To get started and comfortable with intermittent fasting, it's best to do it on a weekly or monthly basis. Even an occasional fasting session gives you a lot of benefits, so you might want to take advantage of it, not just to cut down on calories, but for a healthier lifestyle. For instance — if lunch on Monday is your last meal of the day, you fast until Tuesday's lunch. Seems daunting, but it is actually easy. This schedule allows you to eat each day, at the same time, while still reaping the advantages of a 24 hour fast. You will only cut down on two meals per week, so this is a great option if you're looking to bulk up or keep your weight constant. The biggest benefit of this method is that it helps you overcome your mental barriers with regards to fasting. For people who have never fasted before and those who are apprehensive about taking it up, this is a great way to begin.

Alternate Day Intermittent Fasting

This method incorporates longer fasting periods, but not on consecutive days. For instance — you have your dinner on Monday evening, not eat anything until Tuesday evening, and eat all day on Wednesday. You begin the 24 hour fasting cycle again on Wednesday night. This method helps you fast on a consistent basis, while retaining the calorie count and giving you nutrition. It is also the method of choice for various research studies, providing reliable, scientifically sound evidence showcasing the benefits that it can bring you, which can make taking the leap into fasting less frightening.

The best part about this method is that it gives you a longer fasting period than any of the other methods, thus increasing the amount of time your body needs to burn fat as fuel. But make sure you eat enough when you are in a non-fasting stage, as that is the fuel your body will burn during the fasting period. Teaching yourself to eat on a constant basis needs time and practice. Learning to feast at every meal is not easy, and takes a lot of planning and eating what you have cooked. What this method does is this — people end up losing weight because even though the number of meals reduces, the quantity remains the same.

The calorie ingestion takes place normally. For people looking to lose weight or get leaner, this method is not difficult to follow. But if you are planning to fast for 24 hours per day, on multiple days of the week, it will prove to be extremely difficult to stick to this method. Therefore, it is prudent to try intermittent fasting on a weekly basis first, and try this method only after you get used to it.

Intermittent fasting is a type of partial fasting that isn't as hard as total fasts and can actually help you lose fat and build muscle. How? Read on.

James-Sinclair

Chapter 2

What is Intermittent Fasting and How Does It Work?

Many people see intermittent fasting as a diet but it isn't. Instead, it is more of a dieting pattern, a conscious decision that you make to skip specific meals. By consciously and purposely fasting and then feasting, you are eating your allocated calories inside of a certain window, a certain part of the day and then choosing not to have anything to eat for the rest. Before your eyes light up with the thought of being able to stuff your face in that window of time, there are a couple of things you need to keep in mind:

·   Pick a time span and regularly eat during that

specific time. For example, some people opt for a four or a six-hour window, and some will choose to only eat between the hours of 1 pm to 9 pm, which means not eating any breakfast. Any time window is fine, but it is important for you to be consistent.

· On one day, skip out on two meals, which means you will be going a full day with no food. If you normally have your evening meal at 7 pm, don't eat anything again until 7 pm the next evening.

Now, I can see your brain ticking here. You're thinking that, by skipping out on a meal, you are eating less than you would normally and that means that you will instantly lose weight. Partly, although weight loss is never instant. By cutting one meal a day, you can eat more at the other meals and still eat fewer calories than you would normally, which should lead to a weight loss. However, we all know that not all calories are the same — let's say an apple and a biscuit have the same amount of calories. By eating the apple, not only are you getting the benefits of fiber, you will feel fuller for longer. Eat the biscuit and you are eating sugar, saturated fat and all sorts of other taboo foods. And let's face it, one biscuit leads to another...and another...and before you know it, you've eaten half the packet. So, it isn't always all about **how much** you eat, rather it's about **what** you eat.

How Does Intermittent Fasting Work?

Intermittent fasting isn't some sort of mumbo jumbo or a senseless fad which has recently cropped up. It is based on sound scientific studies and research and throws light on many misconceptions surrounding it. A recent study by the University of Southern California has found that fasting for just three days can reboot and boost your entire immune system. This method proves to be amazing because you reap the benefits of a traditional fast without feeling deprived or weak or faint.

Go online and you will find blogs written about this new style of fasting, which provides fat loss, muscle gain, increased stamina, greater gains at the gym, improved focus and superior immune health, not to mention the previously discussed mental health and discipline improvements. A study published in the Nutrition Journal concluded that calorie restriction and intermittent fasting worked wonders in helping obese people cut their bad fat and lower their risk of cardiovascular disease. Of course, as with any new technique or diet, intermittent fasting does seem to have its drawbacks. The American Journal of Clinical Nutrition found that the alternate day fasting plan could decrease or deplete the glucose levels and interfere with your metabolism. Some women reported increased hunger pangs, higher blood pressure and elevated levels of LDL and HDL in their blood, which is potentially dangerous.

With intermittent fasting, your body works differently when you are fasting than when you are feasting. When you eat, your body takes a few hours out to process the meal. It burns what it can as energy. Because your meal has given your body all of this readily available energy to use, it is going to touch what you have got stored and, what it can't burn is then directed into those stores, building up. This is truer if your meal is made up of sugars and carbohydrates as your body chooses sugar, or glucose, as its primary source of energy.

When you fast, your body hasn't got that meal to convert into energy and, as such, it needs to turn to the fat stores for energy instead of sugar in the bloodstream or the glycogen that is stored in the liver and the muscles. So that's a win right there — burning fat instead of sugar. The same thing goes for when you work out during a fast. Because your body doesn't have that supply of glycogen and glucose (because it has all been depleted during the fast) it has to adapt and take its energy from an alternative source — the fat stores in your cells.

Think of it this way. Say you're 5 years old and you're at the dinner table. Your parents are trying to make you eat spinach for your health but you don't want to be a Popeye. On the table are pot roast, fried chicken and or course, spinach. Because you love anything that isn't spinach, you go for the pot roast first. Next evening, your parents didn't cook you any more food but only prepared last night's leftovers — fried chicken and spinach. Of course, you didn't go for the spinach and went after the fried chicken instead. Next evening, your parents did the same again. So all you had left was spinach. You're darn hungry you could eat a horse — any kind of horse. In this case, spinach is the only horse left for you to eat. Since you're desperate to end your hunger, you eat the spinach. You didn't finish it so your dinner the following evening was the leftover spinach. You eventually ate it as last resort.

In a sense, that's how intermittent fasting helps you lose body fat. By depleting your pot roasts and fried chickens (carbs and glycogen), your body is forced to consume body fat (spinach, the last resort) for energy. You effectively teach your body to increasingly rely on your stored body fat for energy. And the more it does, guess what? You become closer and closer to being ripped.

So, why does this work? When you eat, your body reacts to all that free energy by creating a hormone called insulin. If your body is sensitive to insulin, the food you eat will be consumed far more efficiently, leading to the creation of muscle mass and the loss of body fat. Due to building up a tolerance and therefore effectively becoming used to process insulin when you eat regular, multiple meals each day, your body loses its natural sensitivity to insulin. But that sensitivity can be regained. Your body is going to be more sensitive to this hormone just after a time of fasting, and the results will be more notable as you progressively adjust to your new fasting lifestyle.

When you sleep or fast, the glycogen that is stored in the liver and muscles is gradually depleted and, if you work out, it will be even further depleted, and that increases your insulin sensitivity. When you eat a meal after a period of fasting, it is stored in a more efficient way, most of it going to the muscles as glycogen, burned off as energy straight away to help your body in the recovery process and very little of it going to the fat stores.

Now compare that to a normal day in your life. Your sensitivity to insulin is at a normal level, the food you eat, the carbohydrates in particular, will replenish your glycogen stores, there will be plenty of glucose in your blood and that makes it all more likely that your fat stores will fill to overflowing as well.

When you sleep or after a period of fasting, the secretions of growth hormone increase in your body and insulin production decreases. This results in a higher sensitivity to insulin, which means that you are priming your body to burn fat and increase muscle mass with intermittent fasting. In short, intermittent fasting helps your body to learn how to utilize what food it gets in a more efficient way.

Why Intermittent Fasting?

Because it works, it's as simple as that. We know that calories are all different and we know that restricting calories plays a big role in losing weight. If you fast for 16 hours every day or 24 hours every couple of days, you are automatically restricting how many calories you take in throughout the week. This gives your body a chance to shed a few pounds in a relatively easy way.

Unlike the misconception shared by many, intermittent fasting is a pattern of eating and *not* a diet. It involves organizing your meals so that you can derive the very best out of them. Intermittent fasting doesn't necessarily change the things you eat, as it generally only changes the times you eat. It cuts out the need to go on a strict, low- to no-calorie diet and still offers you a great way to maintain a healthy weight and keep your muscle mass intact.

Also, it makes your day simple. Instead of having to make and pack up food to eat every few hours, you only have to worry about what you eat in your window of time. It takes up less time and you save money in the long run, because you do not have to buy the food to make up three to six meals a day, only two. Instead of stopping what you are doing to eat, you skip a meal and don't stop. Instead of having to wash up three to six lots of dishes, you are only doing two.

Most people get into intermittent fasting in order to get rid of extra pounds. Fortunately, it truly is one of the easiest ways for eliminating bad weight and maintaining a healthy weight since it involves minimal behavioral changes. This implies that intermittent fasting is actually simple enough for you to do, and valuable enough to make a difference.

Intermittent fasting also promotes a stronger sensitivity to insulin and increases growth hormones, which are both key to losing weight and gaining muscle mass. And the more muscle mass you have, the higher your metabolism, which results in fat burning off much quicker and food being utilized better. Intermittent fasting means you win all the way around.

Myths Regarding Intermittent Fasting

As is the case with diets and nutrition, intermittent fasting too has its share of myths and misconceptions. Read on and do not fall prey to them.

Myth 1:

Intermittent fasting will help you lose body fat without undergoing a calorie deficit.

Explanation: When you go without food for long periods of time, your body starts burning fat as fuel. Fasting also increases your insulin sensitivity levels, which further help in storing less fat. So, it would seem as if you can lose fat by fasting for a few hours, and build muscle while you are eating. The problem with this idea is simple — your total caloric intake for the day evens out gradually. If you eat enough during your feed times, you will replace the body fat lost during the fasting state. Studies have also been conducted which clearly show that there is no strong evidence to support the theory that intermittent fasting will help you lose your body fat without a calorie deficit. If you wish to lose weight, you need to eat less than you burn.

Myth 2:

Intermittent Fasting is detrimental to your health

Some people believe that fasting is absolutely injurious to the health, but that's a wrongly preconceived notion. On the contrary, intermittent fasting has remarkable health benefits, according to recent studies. From protection against diseases to maintaining good brain health, intermittent fasting positively affects the state of a person's wellbeing. It can also reduce risk factors for heart disease, inflammation, and oxidative stress and can help boost insulin sensitivity.

Myth 3:
Intermittent fasting will help you lose body fat and build muscle at the same time.

Explanation: There is almost no scientific evidence that supports this theory. Of course, intermittent fasting does help you lose weight, but that is only during the period where you are in a fasting state. Moreover, if you adopt the alternate day intermittent fasting method, you will lose less muscle mass than if you adopt the daily method. A complete beginner or novice would do well to first try out the alternate method. That will help him or her to lose body fat and build lean muscle, but not at the same time.

Myth 4:
Intermittent fasting is a form of starving

One of the most common contentions against intermittent fasting is that it's a way of starving and depriving your body of food, which shuts down your metabolism and hinders fat-burning. Although it's true that prolonged weight loss can decrease the number of calories burned, this is common to weight loss regardless of the method you use. It has not been proven that this is more associated with intermittent fasting than with other weight loss techniques. As a matter of fact, there is substantial evidence that short-term fasting can improve the rate of metabolism due to a dire surge in norepinephrine levels in the blood. The bottom line is, fasting, especially for short periods, does not send the body into starvation. Rather, for fasts lasting up to 48 hours, metabolism is boosted by the fast.

Myth 5:
Intermittent fasting is a suitable alternative to snacking throughout the day.

Explanation: People will keep telling you different things. Eat six or seven small meals a day. Or eat three large ones and two small ones. Go on a juice only diet. Self-styled dietitians go around advocating these lines to people who are desperate to lose weight. Nowadays, the trend is reversing, with diet books proclaiming that a large number of small meals per day is not good for the health. But to each his own. If you find that such an arrangement suits your health requirements, by all means, go for it. Snacking on unhealthy food items in the day is the result of constant hunger brought on by unwise diets. Intermittent fasting is not a diet. It is simply the rearrangement of your eating schedules. You do get to eat good, wholesome food whenever you sit down for a meal, only the meal frequency changes. Therefore, intermittent fasting is by no means an alternative to snacking.

Myth 6:
Intermittent Fasting Makes You Overeat

Another unfounded claim about intermittent fasting is that it instigates over-eating during eating periods. This is partly correct, as people tend to eat a bit more instinctively during a fast to compensate for the lost calories. However, this doesn't paint a complete picture. For instance, a certain study revealed that subjects who were involved in a whole day's fast ate about 500 additional calories the next day. During the fast, they burned off about 2400 calories and over-consumed the extra 500 calories the next day. This means that the net reduction in calorie intake was 1900 which is quite substantial for only two days and proves that intermittent fasting helps you lose weight and not gain it. It is surely one of the most potent tools for weight loss. Implying that intermittent fasting makes you overeat and gain weight could not be further from the truth.

Myth 7:
Women should not undergo intermittent fasting.

Explanation: There is some scientific evidence behind the theory that women don't respond as well to fasting as much as men do. One study found that alternate intermittent fasting decreased the glucose tolerance levels in women and their ability to process sugar. It also made them hungrier and more likely to cheat on the schedule. Yet there is no evidence that intermittent fasting is dangerous for women. Additional studies have shown than while certain women display negative reactions to such a fasting state, it works just fine with other women. It is simply a question of individual constitution and will power, and of course, not all nutrition choices, no matter how beneficial, work equally well for everyone. No matter what your gender, you can, with the right mindset, manufacture an intermittent fasting schedule that works for your body and health needs. Whether you're a woman is not the question at all.

Myth 8:

Intermittent Fasting will slow down your metabolism

Another common half-truth regarding intermittent fasting is that it ultimately slows down your metabolism. There's a grain of truth in that. When you fast, or your body goes without receiving nourishment, your metabolic rate is lowered as a survival technique to prolong survival. Yet, it's important to keep in mind that this only happens when you go without food for more than a week. In fact, one study revealed that in subjects that fasted for three days, there was no slowdown in their metabolism. Plus, intermittent fasting does not involve fasting for that long, therefore, thinking that your body and metabolism will grind to a standstill is unfounded. Understandably, this worry is logical because a slower metabolism is every dieter's worst nightmare. However, as already explained, such worries and fears lack basis, because fasting is not dieting.

Chapter 3

Benefits of Intermittent Fasting

Intermittent fasting has plenty of benefits, one of which is to help you to lose weight. However, there is no magic here, it isn't a quick weight loss formula and, just because you may choose to fast a couple of times per week, it doesn't mean that you can gorge out on junk for the rest of the week. That is the quickest way to fill your body with rubbish and to increase the amount of calories you eat. This leads to weight gain and the misguided assumption that intermittent fasting is not effective, when, like any nutritional plan, it's all about what food you allow into your body. The following 10 benefits of intermittent fasting are firmly based on solid evidence:

It changes the way your hormones, genes and cell function

When you don't eat anything for several hours, a number of things begin to happen in your body. One of the most important things that happens is that your body begins a series of processes that repair your cells and change your hormone levels so that the stored body fat is easier to get at. Some of those changes include:

· Levels of insulin in your blood drop significantly, which helps with the fat burning process

· The levels of human growth hormone in your blood increase by as much as 5 times. These higher levels help the fat burning process, muscle gain and other benefits besides

· The body begins to repair its cells and remove waste material that has built up in them

· Some genes and molecules, particularly those related to disease protection and longevity, start to change

Most of the benefits to intermittent fasting are hormone-related, as well as benefiting both gene and cell function.

It can help you to drop pounds and lose fat from your belly

Most people who choose to try intermittent fasting are doing it because they want to lose some weight. Simply put, intermittent fasting means that you are eating fewer meals and, provided you don't make up for it when you do eat, you will be eating less calories. As well as that, intermittent fasting boosts the function of your hormones, which leads to more effective use of your food and to weight loss.

Lower levels of insulin, higher levels of growth hormones and more norepinephrine in your body all contribute to body fat breaking down and being used as an energy source. Because of this, intermittent, short-term fasting will increase your metabolism by up to 14%, which allows you to burn off more calories without even really trying. In simple terms, intermittent fasting will work on both sides — it boosts your metabolism, which is an increase in calories out of your body while cutting down the amount of food you are eating, resulting in a decrease in calories in. According to a review of scientific literature in 2014, intermittent fasting can be responsible for an incredible weight loss of between 3 and 8% over the course of 3 to 24 weeks.

The people who took part in the research also lost an incredible 4 to 7% of the circumference of their waistline, indicating that quite large amounts of belly fat were lost — fat stored in the abdominal cavity is a particularly harmful type of fat storage, as well as being a prime spot that many of us desire to look fit and toned in.

It reduces your resistance to insulin, lowering the risk of type 2 diabetes

Type 2 diabetes has become very common in the last few decades. The main cause of higher than normal levels of blood sugar, indicating a high resistance level. Anything that can help to lower your resistance will also lower the levels of sugar in your blood and that is one of the biggest protectors against type 2 diabetes. Intermittent fasting has been shown to benefit insulin resistance vastly and can lead to a very significant drop in glucose levels. Studies carried out on humans have shown that fasting blood sugar can be reduced by as much as 6%. While fasting insulin is down by between 20 and 31%. A study that was carried out on diabetic rats also showed that intermittent fasting could help to protect against kidney damage, which is one of the biggest complications in diabetes.

What this means in real terms is that intermittent fasting could be very beneficial to those who are of a higher risk level of type 2 diabetes. However, there is a difference in genders, which must be kept in mind. A study on women showed that the levels of blood sugar actually got worse after a 22-day protocol of intermittent fasting. Consider discussing the risks and benefits with your doctor or medical provider if you are at an increased risk for contracting type 2 diabetes.

It positively affects your cells and hormones

Fasting triggers different changes in your body both on the molecular and cellular level. For instance, hormone levels become altered to provide more access to stored body fat. Also, cells change gene expression and start critical repair processes. A summary of these changes include:

Insulin: The level of insulin drops noticeably as insulin sensitivity increases. This makes stored fat more available.

Human Growth Hormone (HGH): Intermittent fasting can spike the levels of growth hormone to about five times its normal levels. This is beneficial for muscle gain and fat loss.

Gene expression: Genes undergo changes in their functions to act more in disease protection and longevity.

Cellular Repair: Your cells start numerous repair processes on a cellular level during fasting. A typical example is an autophagy, which involves the digestion and removal of useless proteins that are built up in the cells.

These cellular processes in totality are responsible for the various health benefits associated with intermittent fasting.

It reduces inflammation and oxidative stress in your body

One of the biggest factors in premature aging and a high number of chronic diseases is oxidative stress. Unstable molecules that you know of as free radicals react with DNA, protein and other important molecules, causing them damage. Intermittent fasting has been shown to increase your body's resistance to oxidative stress and it can also help to fight off inflammation, which is another huge factor in many common diseases.

It may be beneficial to the health of your heart

The biggest killer in the world right now is heart disease. There are a number of risk factors involved in the risk of someone being more or less likely to be a victim of heart disease and intermittent fasting has been shown to combat many of those factors, including bad cholesterol (LDL), blood pressure, total cholesterol, inflammatory markers, triglycerides, and glucose levels.

That said, a lot of this research has been carried out on animals rather than humans, although much work is being carried out on researching the same factors in humans.

It induces repair processes at a cellular level

During a fast, the body begins to remove waste products from cells. This means that the cells break down and metabolize any dysfunctional or broken proteins that have built up inside them over time. This process is known as autophagy and an increase in it can help to protect against some cancers, Alzheimer's, and many other diseases.

It can be useful to maintain healthy weight

One of the most popular reasons why people go into

intermittent fasting is weight loss. Fortunately, fasting involves eating fewer meals and results in a visible reduction in the number of calories consumed. Plus, intermittent fasting affects hormonal levels to promote weight loss by releasing noradrenaline (norepinephrine) which is the hormone responsible for burning fat. Your metabolic rate also becomes much increased, which is a required precursor for weight loss. The most important thing to remember is that all this can only work if you consume fewer overall calories. Eating excessively and binging during meal periods may nullify your weight loss goal.

It may help to prevent some cancers

Cancer is one of the worst diseases in the world and comes in many different forms, all of them characterized by one thing — the uncontrolled growth of the cells. Intermittent fasting has conclusively shown, on animals and on humans, to have a number of effects, all of them beneficial, on the metabolism. This may lead to a lower risk of cancer. It has also been shown, from studies carried out on humans, that fasting could help to reduce some of the side effects of chemotherapy.

It's good for your brain

It's well known that, if something is good for your body, it is generally good for your brain, too. Intermittent fasting has been shown to improve metabolic function and this is known to be good for the health of your brain. Oxidative stress is reduced; inflammation is reduced, as are the resistance to insulin and the levels of glucose in the blood.

Research has also shown that intermittent fasting can increase the rate at which new nerve cells grow, and increases the levels of BDNF — brain-derived neurotropic factor. This is fully implicated in the chances of a person suffering from depression, as well as a number of other problems with the brain. And intermittent fasting has also been shown to protect you against damage to the brain from strokes.

It may help to prevent Alzheimer's disease

Alzheimer's is the leading neurodegenerative disease in the world and is the most common one. Right now, there isn't a cure for this terrible disease and that means it is more important than ever to look at preventing it in the first place. Intermittent fasting has been shown to delay the onset of Alzheimer's in some people, and reduce the severity of it in others. It has also been shown to protect against many other neurodegenerative brain disease, including Huntington's and Parkinson's.

It simplifies your healthy lifestyle

It's common knowledge that eating healthy is simple. Still, there's no denying that sticking to healthy meals every day can be incredibly stressful, especially when you think of all the work involved to plan and prepare a healthy dish. Intermittent fasting simplifies this process because it crosses out the need to prepare and cook as much as you used to. For this reason, it is very popular because it makes your life easier while improving your health at the same time.

It may help to extend your life

It's no secret that a lower calorie intake is a scientifically proven way of prolonging life, and it makes sense from a logical standpoint. When you starve, your body immediately seeks ways of extending your life. The only thing is, why would anyone go into starvation mode just to live longer? It sure doesn't sound appealing or appetizing in any way. Fortunately, intermittent fasting gives you the benefits of longevity minus the stress of starving. This is because, like calorie restriction, intermittent fasting triggers the exact mechanisms for prolonging life.

Longevity is probably one of the most exciting of all the benefits of intermittent fasting. At this stage, the studies have only been carried out on rats but they show that, in rats that fasted on alternate days, life span was increased by 83% over those that did not fast.

Although we are still waiting for the results from human research, those who are interested in anti-aging measures have adopted intermittent fasting vigorously. Given that intermittent fasting has huge metabolic benefits, it makes sense that it can help you live a much healthier and longer life.

You have heard the phrase that a person with great power has great responsibility. If you are someone who is going to start intermittent fasting or are someone who has already started following intermittent fasting, you will need to take care of yourself extremely well. You will need to ensure that you keep yourself healthy; otherwise, you will be harming yourself in ways that will deteriorate your health. I am not trying to scare you off fasting, but asking you to be careful. Let me give you a little information on the detrimental effects of intermittent fasting.

It is much easier than dieting

Starting and sticking to a diet is one of the hardest things to do for most people. Most dieters fail because they cannot continue with a particular diet for an extended time and end up switching to the wrong foods. The crux of the problem is a behavior change problem as opposed to a nutrition problem. In this regard, intermittent fasting takes the upper hand because you get over the conception that you need to eat specific foods (or avoid foods altogether) every time, it becomes amazingly easy to follow. Studies have proven that intermittent fasting is an effective weight-loss approach in obese adults because the subjects adapted quickly to the intermittent fasting regimen.

Intermittent fasting can serve as a helpful travel strategy.

Airports provide a lot of unhealthy food options, and it's almost a herculean task to find a small amount of healthy food in the vicinity. To avoid this problem, you can regard all your travel days as a fasting day. Then the following day, feel free to eat as much healthy food as you'd like!

The Detrimental Effects

There are some detrimental effects of intermittent fasting, which are listed below:

It is easy to create or exacerbate existing eating disorders.

Intermittent fasting, if done to the extreme, can create problems for the body. It can trigger or heighten eating disorders like bulimia and anorexia nervosa. In the feeding state, when one can literally eat anything, people might tend to overeat or binge on unhealthy food items, only to regret it later. This can lead to unhealthy and detrimental behaviors both physically and mentally. You need to be sure you can and will control what you eat in a safe and healthy way during your feeding periods to avoid creating a harmful self-image and either fasting too much or purging after your eating times, both of which are very harmful to your health. People with an already existing eating disorder should first get treated for their problem before embarking on intermittent fasting.

You may be uncomfortably full after eating

Most people are used to eating several times every day. This eating pattern makes it possible to consume sufficient amounts of food without feeling too full at any given time. In the case where you have a small window for eating, you would need to wolf down one or two large meals which can result in you feeling constipated and uncomfortable. Also, having big meals for dinner before you go to bed can prevent you from having a good night sleep.

When the fasting period ends, you'll feel ravenous and end up eating a lot of food. Then a few hours before you begin your fast, you'll eat again. This means that if you want to try intermittent fasting, you would need to be able to handle large meals and be okay with having a stretched-out stomach for a couple of hours. Plus, digesting a large meal can unduly stress out the body.

Your cortisol levels might get chronically elevated, without your knowing it.

When you skip meals, it revs up your stress hormone cortisol, which causes all sorts of havoc on the metabolism. When there is an increase in the amount of cortisol in the short term, the body releases fat as energy. It is dangerous over longer periods of time because fat is no longer used as fuel but stored inside the body and the muscle is used as fuel instead. This leads to burning your muscles for energy that will decrease your fitness level and undermine your efforts. To avoid it, ensure you do not take fasting too far. It is important to eat on a regular basis when practicing intermittent fasting or suffer the hormonal consequences and shoot yourself in the foot.

Food can soon turn into an unhealthy obsession for some.

Picture this — you are into the daily fasting mode and suddenly, you see your friend open her fried chicken lunch across the table. All you can think about now is what you'll have for dinner when you can finally break your fast. Let's face it — hunger is the prime motivator for a great many things. When one's stomach is full, he or she can concentrate on other issues, but when the primary need of hunger is not met for many hours, people become cranky, sullen, angry, and think about food constantly. This can lead to binging during your eating periods, and it can tempt you to cheat and eat when you should still be fasting. It will also encourage you to select unhealthy foods when you do eat, such as sweets, sodas, and greasy fried foods, leading to an overabundance of sugars, bad cholesterol, and saturated fats, thus thwarting the caloric deficit intermittent fasting should entail as well as eliminating the nutrients your body needs for health and well-being. In addition to the physical detriment caused by such behavior, you might become more inclined to snap at or lash out at those around you who are not practicing fasting, harming your interpersonal relationships and your social life, which is highly negative for your mental health. If you struggle to maintain a positive outlook and find yourself giving into temptations, confrontational or other antisocial behavior, or any other thought consuming activities, you might want to alter the intermittent fasting plan that you chose. Fasting for shorter periods of time or easing into it more slowly can lessen resentment and allow your body and mind to adjust to your new commitment in a safe and natural way. The goal here should be for intermittent fasting to become a healthy, normal part of your life and not something you obsess or stress over. If you are prone to the concerns here, start with an easier schedule and take things slow. You will still enjoy many of the benefits while lessening the negative side effects that fasting may have on you.

There might be an over-reliance on caffeine and related products.

Intermittent fasting allows for a generous dose of caffeine and related products, which keep you stimulated and going for hours without the intake actual food or necessary nutrients. This might become a bad habit to break later on. A certain amount of caffeine is okay for the system, but anything beyond three cups of coffee a day will prove to be severely detrimental to both the physical and mental well-being of the person. It disrupts your sleep cycle, elevates your cortisol levels, and may cause you to be alert or nervous. Enjoy your coffee or tea, but do not rely on it as a substitution for food. If you want to sip on a beverage during the day, either for personal enjoyment or as a distraction from hunger, try water. It can work surprisingly well at filling your stomach, and the energy it will give you is safe, natural, and healthy. Even in very high quantities.

Your athletic performance may be greatly impaired

When fasting, mild to moderate workouts are okay. However, participating in intense training and exercises such as cross fit or power lifting can cause more harm than good. According to recent research, fasting leads to a more diminished athletic performance. The athletic performance of runners was tested during a Ramadan fast and during non-fasting periods. It was discovered that the athletes had significantly reduced athletic performance and increased fatigue during fasting than on non-fasting days.

You are at a risk of increased chances of food intolerances and inflammation.

When you fast, you feel famished, and want nothing more than to dive head first into a deep dish pizza or a smoking hot cheeseburger or a sundae when it is time for you to eat. You forget that eating such foods will give a huge boost to your blood sugar levels which will ultimately crash, leaving you feeling lethargic and uneasy. When you do break your fast, it is likely that the foods will contain gluten, dairy, nuts etc. which are all potentially reactive foods, causing inflammation and other gut issues. Therefore, whenever you are in a feeding state, eat sensibly. Instead of binging on comfort food, eat wholesome and naturally occurring food to keep you full and restrict the bad calories you might ingest. This can be difficult to adjust to at first, especially if healthy eating is atypical for you, but ensure you prepare balanced, nutritious, and filling meals for yourself while avoiding trigger foods to ensure the best results possible. You do not have to cut out all imperfect foods and lead a life devoid of flavor, but it is important to ensure sugars and unhealthy fats are used sparsely and to be careful to meet your nutritional needs when you do eat. After all, you will be eating fewer meals to get those nutrients from.

You may now be wondering if you should take up the fast. Do not think too much and give it a shot. Let me give you a picture on how you can start your intermittent fast!

James-Sinclair

Chapter 4

Lessons Learnt from Intermittent Fasting

People who have tried this method of fasting have reported getting stronger and leaner, without giving up their favorite foods and feeling cranky. They have also experienced certain life lessons while undergoing the fasting, some of which are listed below. Look at them as an inspirational guide to get you started on your own journey.

Your mind is your biggest barrier.

If you look at it objectively, this diet is simple to implement. Depending on the kind of fasting you do, you skip certain meals and make up for them at other times.

The biggest hurdle here is telling your mind to accept the changes. People think that if they don't eat at the designated time, they might faint or fall sick. They think that they need to eat every two or three hours, and not skip breakfast at all or have a light dinner. Once you get started on this fasting, you will realize how easy and simple it is, and how much healthier you feel from the inside. It usually helps most people to ease into it slowly. It goes against much of what you have likely been taught and therefore think you know about your body and your health. You will change your mind about that once you see the effects of periodic fasting in action, and over time your fears and apprehensions will be proven to be unfounded. You'll find yourself healthier and more energetic than ever. The hardest part is taking that leap and starting.

It is easy to lose weight and keep it that way.

When the number of calories you ingest is less than the number of calories you burn, you lose weight. It's as simple as that. Intermittent fasting allows one to lose weight without losing muscle mass. It is a great option for people who are looking to lose weight because the weight loss happens without any change in the diet or foods. The only thing which changes is the time when you eat your food. People lose weight with this method because when they eliminate meals from their time plan and they don't binge eat at the next feeding.

It is possible to build muscle while fasting.

People who have tried intermittent fasting have reported gaining lean body mass and cutting body fat by as much as five percent. This happens due to the body's tendency to lose weight during the fasting period. Your body begins to utilize the fat stores you have built up for energy when it does not have readily accessible energy sources from food. But you do not go so long without that your muscle supply becomes fodder for energy. At the end of the day, your caloric intake is the same. Whether you ingest two thousand calories during a 16 hour span or 24 hour span or 8 hour span does not matter. You just need to eat enough to build muscle.

It results in more productivity, at least for some people.

Some people have stated that they experience a lot of mental clarity during their fasting periods. Contrary to popular belief, fasting does not drain the body and mind of energy. Letting go of your focus on and preoccupation with food can enable you to think about and apply your creativity to other interests and activities. No more do you have to consider what you will make for dinner that night and if you have the time. Instead, the day is truly yours, with no need to shop, cook, wash dishes, or even waste your precious time eating. You can focus your mind solely on your interests and desires, as opposed to distracting yourself with something you once thought was a necessity.

Cycling your foods might be the way to go.

Intermittent fasting will work much better when you start cycling your foods and calorie combinations. For instance, eat a bit more when you are going to work out and a bit less when you are on a rest period. This means you will have a calorie surplus on the days you train, and a deficit on the days you rest. By doing this, you build muscle on the days you work out and you burn body fat while you rest. You need to ensure you have the calories and nutrients to use on the days you are working hard in order to gain and keep lean muscle mass. When you want to take it easy and relax, it should be simple enough to just not eat while you do it.

After all, it's nothing more than a mental exercise. You don't physically require the food as much when you are not as active. Your body will just naturally go through your fat stores and you will be closer than ever to achieving your fitness goals and shedding that excess body fat. Keep cycling your carbs and protein with the days you train and rest. This will lead you to become leaner, with elevated muscle mass and low body fat levels.

Take a long term view of eating and dieting, no short cuts here.

The reason most diets don't work out is because we look at them through a very short time frame. Thinking about what you eat over a course of a week is better than tracking what you eat per day. Don't worry about having or not having a protein shake within an hour of working out, especially if you are going to eat a protein rich meal later in the day. This is where intermittent fasting works out better than a conventional diet. For example — you eat three or four wholesome meals in a day, making a total of 21 meals in a week. Do you really think your body cares when the meals are eaten? In a 12 hour schedule or a 16 hour one? Either way, you are ensuring you are getting the calories and nutrients necessary for health and fitness. All you are changing is what times you get them. When you look at things from a long term point of view, you realize that intermittent fasting will ultimately do you good.

When you are in a fasted state, you want less food.

You discover that you are no longer a victim to your diet or food addictions. You eat because you want to eat, not because it's time and you have to eat. This is a marked change from your earlier eating habits and you soon find how beneficial it is to your body and health. You likely will not notice this change at first, as it takes time for your new habits to become your day to day normal, but give it a few weeks, a few months, eventually a few years. The more time passes, the more comfortable and natural fasting will feel and the less you will crave food during your fast days. Additionally, you will likely develop a greater appreciation for eating and enjoy food more when you do eat, because you will be eating because you want to and because you need to, not just because it is a meal time and you feel like you should consume a meal.

You can lose fat and build muscle, but not at the same time.

If you choose a combination of intermittent fasting and calorie cycling, you can lose fat and build muscle with ease. It is physiologically impossible to achieve these two things at the same time. Weight loss involves burning off more calories than you take in. To build muscle, you need to feed your muscle. You obviously can't have a calorie deficit and a caloric surplus at the same time. However, if you take longer time frames into consideration, say a week or a month, then you have better options. For example, if you work out three days a week, you can design your eating plan to include a calorie surplus when you train, and a deficit when you rest. This enables your body to build muscle mass during your eating and training periods, and to focus on burning through fat during your resting and fasting periods. This way, you get the best of both worlds.

You make more gains by training for a lesser amount of time when fasting.

This is how it works — you pick a goal for the week's work out and do the most important and effective exercises first.

Get the compound exercises out of the way. Perhaps upper body in the morning, lower body in the evening. Or pushups in the morning and squats in the evening. Due to the hormonal and metabolic changes you will experience when fasting in this way, your workouts are more effective and your need to train for hours at a time is lessened. People have reported increased gains with this method. Intermittent fasting enables you to see better results with less time spent training for them so it truly is a win-win method.

Drinking lots of water helps. Always.

Intermittent fasting demands that you keep yourself hydrated at all times. Your needs might vary, but a general rule of thumb is to drink around a half a gallon (two liters) of water per day, even if you don't feel like it. Your body only tells you it's thirsty when it is dehydrated. Don't let it reach that state. Normally we obtain some of our water needs from the food we eat, as most foods, especially vegetables and fruits, and rich in water content. You will no longer have this benefit. Drink often. Additionally, it is worth noting that water is surprisingly good at making you feel fuller, lessening your need and desire for daily meals.

There is really no drawback to drinking more water. It's the best possible substance you can consume, and essential for you to achieve your maximum health and fitness potential. Other liquids are okay, but when it comes to fasting and your health, there is no substitute for pure, clean water. Make it a part of your daily routine.

The best diet is the one that works for you and your body.

In this age of short cuts, everyone wants the ultimate diet plan, something written on a piece of paper that will dramatically change their lives and health. This is one reason why diet books sell like hotcakes all year round. People just want a quick fix to their problems. This rarely works, because each person is different. A diet which works for your friend won't necessarily work for you, because the two of you are very different people, with different needs. Your gender, age, body type, and fitness level all are likely to lead to slightly varied plans, not to mention medical conditions or risks, allergies, or any other factors about you, physically or mentally, that might very well alter your perfect diet. You need to experiment and discover what works best for your body. And this is where intermittent fasting scores high. You can play around with your eating schedule and patterns without causing any harm to your body and health. As you experiment you will no doubt find foods and eating schedules that make you feel energetic and spry, as well as those that make you feel more lethargic or otherwise cause negativity in you. Figure out what works for you, and if something doesn't seem ideal, change it. This is one of the wonderful features of intermittent fasting over most other diets. You get to choose when you want to eat what.

Chapter 5

Intermittent Fasting and Exercise

Ever since the first set of weights in the gym were ever lifted, there has been debate about whether it's worse or better to exercise on a stomach with nothing in it. So many friendships have been severed, marriages destroyed, and lives broken as a result of intense debates on this matter of universal importance! Alright, exaggeration aside, this is definitely one of the most controversial topics in the world of health and fitness. In this chapter, you'll settle once and for all this hotly debated topic that has the potential to spark World War III.

One of the things we need to first clear is the concept of

smaller, more frequent meals when it comes to health and fitness. In particular, that doing so is the best way to rev up the metabolism for burning fat and feeding your muscles. Contrary to what most people think is true, there are research results that suggest that this just isn't the case.

Another idea or myth to clear up is that working out on an empty stomach will basically cancel any benefits you may enjoy from working out. Again, some studies have found that that isn't necessarily true. And lastly, the idea that skipping meals will lead to slower metabolism and stronger desire to eat food, which will consequently lead to weight gain also isn't true.

Why do we need to clear those ideas out first? Because those are some of the mindsets or beliefs that aren't consistent with intermittent fasting. Since intermittent fasting is about, well, fasting; exercising on an empty stomach, eating less frequently and skipping "meals" won't make sense to you and you probably won't believe that exercising while fasting intermittently can be beneficial for you.

Hormonal Optimization

Let me offer you proof that intermittent fasting and working out can coexist and coexist well. Friends, let me offer you: Hugh Jackman. In preparing for his most recent Wolverine movie, Jackman got, pardon for the pun, jacked using intermittent fasting. How's that for proof? How'd that happen you might ask?

You see, an empty stomach can help because of hormonal changes inside your body that can foster fat burning and muscle building. In particular, an empty stomach can improve your sensitivity to insulin and increased natural production of growth hormones, which enable you to grow more muscle mass faster.

Your body produces insulin via the pancreas when you eat, which helps you utilize your foods' nutrient content. Insulin removes blood sugar from your blood and drives them to your fat cells, muscles, and liver for future use. The problem usually lies when there is too much — and too often — and as a result, your body may become less sensitive to insulin. Lower insulin sensitivity brings with it a host of other health issues, including inability to lose (or even gain more) body fat and higher risks for cardiovascular diseases and cancer. Eating less frequently — as is the case when you fast intermittently — minimizes your body's production of insulin and as such, lowers your risk for becoming less and less sensitive to it over time. The less insulin your body needs to produce, the more sensitive it becomes to insulin, which helps you burn body fat and lower your risks for diabetes and cardiovascular diseases.

Exercising on an empty stomach also helps your body concoct more of the magical elixir of a hormone called growth hormone or GH, which is important for increasing muscle mass, stronger bones, the ability to burn fat, longevity and improved physical functioning. Some studies have shown that a man's GH production skyrockets by a mesmerizing 2,000% and a woman's by 1,300% when they fast for 24 hours. Could you believe those numbers? All by not eating for 24 hours! And dig this, those studies also showed that as soon as the fast is ended, GH production plummets back down to normal. This is another reason to fast regularly and intermittently — optimal GH production levels.

For men, it's virtually impossible to talk about muscle-building hormones without touching on the big T —

testosterone. It's another magical elixir-of-a-hormone that's responsible for muscle building, fat burning, higher energy levels, elevated libido, and effectively fighting off depression and heart problems. While intermittent fasting itself isn't enough to significantly increase one's T levels, exercising on an empty stomach certainly can.

Supplementation and Resistance Training

Many bodybuilders and fitness buffs are known to be highly dedicated to intermittent fasting. But how do they manage to fast and still maximize their exercise performance? These are some of the best ways to not just achieve your workout goals, but to thrive and optimize while intermittently fasting. These strategies will help replenish energy stores and maximize protein synthesis and recovery.

A Typical Resistance Training Day

Before Workout
Caffeine

Taking a little caffeine before your workout gets you fired up and can significantly increase upper body strength.

Epigallocatechin-3-Gallate (EGCG)

One of the primary goals of intermittent fasting is enhanced fat loss. Therefore, a supplementation goal should be to increase the breakdown of triglycerides or stored fat, through a process known as lipolysis, in addition to fatty acid oxidation (deriving energy from fatty acids). Combining caffeine with EGCG has been shown to significantly increase metabolic rate and fatty acid oxidation.

This blend works together to boost fat loss while regulating the drop in metabolic rate during extended periods of fasting. To increase lipolysis, 150 mg of EGCG should be taken per day. As an alternative, green tea extract (600 – 900mg) can be ingested.

Beta-Alanine

Using beta-alanine as a supplement can help increase your work ability by minimizing fatigue linked to the accumulation of metabolites such as hydrogen ions. A beta-alanine supplement takes effect by raising the levels of an intercellular buffer known as carnosine in the body, which acidity and boosts intense workout performance. to 6.3g of beta-alanine is adequate for daily use.

To administer, split the dosage into three smaller daily servings.

Essential Amino Acids and Carbohydrates

According to certain research, 6g of essential amino acids and 35g of sucrose right before you being intense exercise can extensively increase protein synthesis due to a greater entry of these essential amino acids into the active muscle. The bottom line is, load yourself up with some essential amino acids and 100g of dried dates before hitting the gym to amplify your muscle improvements.

During Workout
Branched-Chain Amino Acids (BCAAS)

Although there's not much extensive research appraising the use of BCAAs during resistance training, their effect is two-fold: 1) decreasing the ratio of BCAA to free tryptophan in the blood and ultimately cutting central fatigue, and 2) preventing slow protein breakdown and boosting recovery. We can therefore safely state that sipping on BCAAs for an entire day can enhance the rate of protein synthesis and help even out some of the protein degradation that may happen during fasting. An effective dose would include 7g of BCAAs with some valine, isoleucine, and leucine.

After Workout

Protein

Protein consumption, for example, like ingesting whey protein before and after you exercise can result in better protein synthesis. About 25g of fat-digesting protein should be immediately consumed after your workout to kick-start the anabolic process.

Carbohydrates

Consuming carbs after your intense training exercise can drastically reduce muscle protein catabolism and restore glycogen levels. A good recommendation would be a workout shake that is loaded with dextrose. However, if snacking on real foods is your preference, it's best to stick to foods like potatoes, rice, pasta or oats.

Creatine

Using creatine supplements of about 4g per day can result in an upsurge of muscle-fiber size, strength, power output and an overall lean body mass. Using creatine after your workout is more efficient than using it before your exercise in terms of strength gains and body composition.

Glutamine

Prolonging the duration, frequency and intensity of your exercise severely affects the level of serum glutamine and has been linked with decreases in immune function. Although there's not enough research on the inhibition of immune setbacks and overtraining in those who participate in body building, ingesting glutamine orally has been discovered to have a substantial effect on the prevention of illness, which is one of the major symptoms of the overtraining syndrome. 10g of L-glutamine can be consumed daily, in two 5g doses. One should be taken right after training, while the other should be ingested two hours after training.

Highway to Performance Improvement

If high intensity compound exercises, i.e., those that involve a large number of muscles and muscle groups, can lead to a significant spike in testosterone levels, doing so while fasting intermittently boosts that spike even further. Studies have shown that working out under a state of fasting is one of the best ways to increase lean muscle mass and improve sensitivity to insulin. This happens due to hormonal responses and the body's ability to absorb more calories after each workout. It goes without saying then that training while fasting intermittently significantly increases the likelihood that fat, protein, and carbohydrate calories go to their respective destinations and minimizes the chances of them being stored as body fat. Instead, the body utilizes them immediately. This will improve your health and build up lean, strong muscle mass.

Exercising on an empty stomach has been found to be especially useful for burning body fat and improving your ability to burn it at higher exercise intensity levels. If the body has sugars available for easy energy right before you exercise, it will use those to provide for its energy needs. No food before you work out? You force your body to target your fat reserves, effectively shedding the weight in even problematic areas and better revealing the muscle mass beneath

.

The Rock?

Are you concerned that you may end up being as bulky as Dwayne "The Rock" Johnson or Dave Batista? Don't worry; those dudes are one in a million. In order to grow at such ginormous dimensions, you need a lot of things, and foremost of which is genetics. And to be honest, only 1% of the planet's total population has the genetics needed to grow as big as them — even with anabolic steroids. So there's no need to worry about getting too big for comfort.

Even if you're not interested in becoming more muscular, exercising while fasting intermittently has other benefits to offer. If you're an endurance athlete, intermittent fasting workouts can help improve your body's efficiency in storing glycogen. In layman's terms, periodically exercising with significantly depleted energy stores can help your body become even more efficient at using its energy stores 24/7.

Occasionally training on an empty stomach can help significantly improve the quality of your non-fasting workouts later on. Bottom line is when your body gets used to exerting itself without food, it'll be able to exert even more with a relatively full tank. Some research reveals that fasted exercise sessions can dramatically increase endurance athletes' capacity to take in and utilize oxygen while exercising, which is a great way to evaluate his or her fitness. In short, exercising on an empty stomach trains your body to perform more efficiently and stronger.

Now, it wouldn't be fair to just present the good side of intermittent fasting exercise. There are studies that have also shown that physical exercises while fasting can lead to poorer performance. It's worth noting though, that these studies were done during Ramadan involving Muslims. If you're not very familiar with the Islamic religion, Ramadan is a very important religious period where Muslims are called to fast every day and their fast prohibits them even from drinking water, which is a very important part of any exercise session for that matter. It is very important to listen to your body and be aware of the improvements, or lack thereof, that occurs with your performance. If you are careful to stay well hydrated, though, research suggests that you have much to gain.

I assume that upon reaching this point in this book, you're still sold on the idea of achieving a ripped, muscular condition via intermittent fasting and working out while doing so. I also assume you're willing to start doing it already as soon as you finish this book. That being said, what should you do as you start your exercise plan while intermittently fasting?

Where the Rubber Meets the Road

You may now be starting to think about how hard and torturous exercising on an empty stomach can be. This is the part where I'll tell you to give yourself more credit. You can do it and it's important that you believe you can because your "I believe I can" is more important than your "I can."

One of the reasons you may be thinking negatively, if ever, is fear of the unknown. In that case, I'll help you reduce the unknowns with the following tips in order to reduce your fears about starting to work out on an empty stomach.

More Than Just Water

To help you power through your workouts, especially during the first few, don't hesitate to drink more than just water. You may include pure green tea, pure black coffee, caffeine pills, creatine, or just about any performance enhancing supplements that are practically calorie free. There are also a number of vitamins (think any of the B types primarily) as well as herbal teas and supplements that are virtually devoid of calories and can work wonders for boosting your energy level in a natural, relatively safe manner.

All-Day Break (the) Fast

You can break your fast at any time of the day that you like. For many, they intentionally schedule their first meal or their workouts in such a way that their first meal is right after working out. This is because anything you eat within the so-called post exercise golden window (within 3 hours after working out) has very little chance of being stored as body fat, thereby maximizing the fat loss benefits of exercising on an empty stomach.

If you prefer to exercise first thing in the morning and have your first meal at night, no worries. The spike in GH production from working out on an empty stomach should be more than enough to prevent muscle loss — also known as muscle catabolism — during the day. It's now really up to you.

Eating Frequency

You can eat as many meals as you like, which is a whole lot

different from taking in as many calories as you want. Contrary to popular belief, your body can digest all your day's requirement in one meal, which doesn't necessarily mean you should consume only one meal. Just because you can doesn't mean you should, right?

There's no conclusive evidence showing that eating smaller and more frequent meals is significantly better at helping you either shed fat or build muscle compared to eating bigger but less frequent meals. It may take a lot longer to fully digest the amount of protein you eat in fewer yet bigger meals but the bottom line is that it will still be digested. The key is to experiment with different meal sizes and frequencies (check out the protocols later) to see what will work best for you.

The Bottom Line

As humans, we are generally creatures of habit and the way we eat is one of the most ingrained habits we all have. As such, eating less frequently may be a very challenging task to accomplish at first, especially if you're a very healthy eater. But don't worry — all habits take time to break and replace. It's been said that habits — on average — take 21 straight days of practicing before becoming, well, a habit. If it's been significantly longer than that, don't be afraid to conclude that it may not be for you. It's better to have tried than forever be thinking "what if?" Remember, intermittent fasting is just one of the many approaches to health and fitness. There is one out there that's right for you should this one not pan out.

However, allow me to say this before I end this chapter: there really is no need to eat before working out. Even if you decide that intermittent fasting does not work for you, a good take away message from this book would be to at least try out exercising on an empty stomach for a while and see how it works out for you. But if you feel better eating prior, nothing is stopping you and no police will apprehend you for doing so. Just keep it to a minimum and avoid stuffing yourself prior in order to actually burn fat and avoid puking while working out.

Chapter 6

Building Muscle...Fast(ing)

Many people have managed to actually gain weight even while on intermittent fasting, most of which was muscle. It's because intermittent fasting isn't necessarily about cutting down on your total daily caloric intake — though that would be the case if your primary reason for doing it were shedding off body fat — but about cutting down on frequency of eating. In other words, those who have gained more muscle mass while on intermittent fasting focused on increasing total daily caloric intake during their daily feeding windows. This is not a recommendation to binge eat during your feeding windows. It is simply about choosing healthy, nutritious, and yes, highly caloric foods when you do eat in order to enable your body to gain your desired muscle mass.

The reason why people naturally equate intermittent fasting with fat or weight loss is because of the natural tendency to eat fewer calories when you cut out a meal or two daily. But as I mentioned earlier, intermittent fasting is more about meal frequency and spacing, not total calories. So in order to build muscle, you simply need to consume more calories daily and you can still do that even if you limit your eating frequency or period. Simply consume all your daily caloric needs within the remaining number of meals or eating period that you have allotted to yourself. Apart from having to go on an empty stomach for longer, the other challenge would be to eat more than the usual amount of food per meal or within your eating window. As such, you can still gain muscle, if so desired, while on an intermittent fast. Remember Hugh Jackman? Right!

As a result, more and more people are starting to become curious about intermittent fasting in general and in the different protocols in particular. The choice of which particular protocol to follow all boils down to one's lifestyle and daily schedule. Some have more time to follow the more time consuming protocols while others have less time available so the simpler but harder protocols may be just what the nutritionist and trainer ordered for them. More than the schedule, another aspect of lifestyle is religion. Muslims, for example, are required to fast daily from 5 in the morning to 7 in the evening during Ramadan. If your reasons for trying out intermittent fasting are one part fitness and health, one part religion or spirituality, rest assured that the two can go hand and hand and there are plenty of fantastic plan choices that should work for you.

Regardless of your circumstances, you can practice intermittent fasting and incorporate a great workout regimen that will allow you to build more muscle and eventually, reduce your overall body fat. This is because muscle cells are metabolically active, i.e., the more of it you have, the faster your metabolism becomes.

The following are guidelines to help you successfully build muscle while fasting intermittently.

The Later, The Better

If like the Muslims, you choose a specific time period for fasting daily like the Ramadan-prescribed 5 a.m. to 7 p.m.

schedule, you'd be well off to schedule your exercise or workout sessions late in the evening or even during the early morning. Doing so helps you to get your nutrients in before and after working out, especially if you're talking about lifting weights. You can have your first meal by 7 p.m. and an hour or two after, hit the weights, and eat a recovery meal before hitting the sack say at 10 p.m. Then you can wake up before 5 a.m. to have another meal to power you through the rest of the day so by the time 5 a.m. rolls in, you've already replenished much needed nutrients and are fully charged for the day. This gives you, assuming a wakeup call of around 4 o'clock a.m., a six-hour feeding period each day. You can tweak this plan to take every other day off eating as well, especially as you become more experienced and comfortable with intermittent fasting. Do a total fast one day, 6 hour eating period the next.

Post Workout Emphasis

In attempting to build muscle while fasting intermittently, the wisest way for you to apportion your daily calories is by consuming the biggest chunk of your calories during your post-workout meal. The reason for this is post-workout recovery and calories consumed during the 3-hour golden post-workout window tend to be used more efficiently by the body, e.g., for building muscle instead of being stored as fat.

That being said, you'll need to figure out just how many calories you need to build muscle and consume about 20% of that prior to exercising or working out. Take in a good mixture of carbs and protein. Then as soon as you end your workout, consume about 60% of your calories right after your workout and prior to hitting the sack. If it's too much for you to eat all at once, consider spreading it out over 2 to 3 meals within the next 2 to 4 hours before hitting the sack.

Taking in 60% of your daily caloric requirements may seem too much to take in a relatively short span of time, and frankly it can be intimidating. If you find that after several days you're still having a hard time doing so, then consider eating foods that are calorie dense, i.e., contain more calories per gram such as dried fruits, red meat, bagels, and raw oats, among others, in order for you to meet the requirement. Since calorie dense foods have packed significantly more calories, you can actually eat less in terms of volume and still meet your 60% target. Be sure to select nutritious food, though. It can be easy to fall into the trap of choosing bacon, cookies, and other junk food in order to pack in a lot of calories in a relatively small amount of time, but you'll not do yourself or your fitness level any favors by making poor decisions. Jerky, nuts, fruit juice with no sugar added. There are a lot of delicious, health conscious choices you can make when breaking your fast.

Given that you're going to be consuming the bulk of your daily calories after working out, you'd be better off going higher carb and lower fat than low carbs and high fat. This is because for post workout recovery, carbs are better than fat. They are the fastest and easiest energy form to digest and the most natural energy source you can provide to your body. Just take note that low fat doesn't mean no fat. Just keep it to at most 15% of total daily calories. And because fat is the most calorie dense among the 3 major macronutrients at 9 calories per gram compared to only 4 calories per gram each for carbs and protein, high fat foods can be a good way to reduce the volume of food you need without scrimping on calories. Choose nuts, nut butters, seeds, healthy cuts of meat, and other nutritional sources of fat and you can enjoy a very decent, high calorie meal that you might actually be able to consume in a single sitting.

Eat as Soon as You Wake Up

Lastly, it's best that you eat something right after your natural waking up time when fasting intermittently. If you're sticking to the 5 a.m. to 7 p.m. fasting period Ramadan-style, it means making sure you eat something before 5 a.m. In particular, go for slow-digesting protein that can help you feel fuller for longer and help keep your body in an anabolic state, i.e., muscle building state, for longer during the day even without eating. These food items include red meat and cottage cheese, which should make up the remaining 20% of your daily caloric requirements.

While it's not a bad idea to throw in some carbs into the meal, limit the amount so that you get at least 35% of your daily protein calorie requirements from this meal, which is crucial to maintaining an anabolic state throughout the day. Do this with the goal of consuming only 20% of your total daily caloric requirements for this meal.

Don't Scrimp On the Calories

If you're doing relatively higher intensity or volume workout sessions, just make sure you consume enough calories to power such workouts. While you can sustain such workouts with low calories and intermittent fasting, it won't be long before it catches up on you and you burn out. It's impossible because over time, your glycogen stores will be depleted and your workouts and recovery will be severely compromised. Your muscular gains will cease and your body will eventually begin to burn through the muscle you already have, leading to muscular atrophy and poorer health overall. As such, you'll need to learn to eat more food within a smaller time period and less eating frequency to ensure you get enough calories to build muscle. It's a good idea to take your time and ease into the change. Start slowly. Over time, you'll adjust to it and it'll feel natural to you.

Chapter 7

Top Intermittent Fasting Protocols

These six methods of intermittent fasting all take advantage of the huge benefits gained but everyone who tries it will find that some methods work better for them than others. At the end of the day, we are all different and our bodies will respond to different things. Don't force yourself to continue with a protocol that is clearly not working. Instead, give another one a try. Find the method that makes life easier for you, not more difficult. Otherwise, it simply won't be a sustainable way of life and you will very quickly fall back into your old ways.

Each of these protocols comes with its own set of guidelines on how long you should fast for and what you should focus on eating during your feeding window. Here, I am going to give you a basic overview of how each method works, along with its pros and cons. Do keep in mind that intermittent fasting may not work for everyone and, if you have any kind of health or medical issues, you need to speak with your physician before you start making any changes to your diet or meal schedule.

Leangains

Leangains is an intermittent fasting based diet and training style authored by Martin Berkhan which has grown immensely popular in the last 5 years. To be more specific, Leangains may be considered a program for improving one's body composition, i.e., body fat levels, using an intermittent fasting diet that cycles carbohydrates and a training program based on power bodybuilding. It may sound so technical and complicated but really, it isn't. In simpler terms, Leangains is a diet and training program aimed at helping you achieve your best body fat and lean muscle levels.

You can use the Leangains program to achieve any of the

three body composition goals: get cut; bulk up; or recomposition. When we say getting cut, I don't mean wounded, right?   I mean losing as much body fat as possible while retaining as much of your physical strength and lean muscle mass as possible. Bulking up doesn't mean gaining weight and size for the simple reason of doing so but to gain lean muscle mass and consequently, strength, with minimal increase in body fat. Recomposition means to improve your ratio of lean muscle mass to body fat gradually over the course of time.

Truth be told, this program isn't rocket science or as complicated as calculus. Its main goal is to lift weights 2 to 3 times every week, focusing on compound exercises, i.e., involving as many muscle groups in one exercise as possible, most of the time. If needed, supplemental works are added. The program emphasizes minimalism, which is great especially for very busy people whose time is limited.

How it Works

Women should fast for a 14-hour period, men for a 16-hour period each day. Your feeding window is a set time of eight to ten hours. While you are fasting, you must consume nothing that has any calories in it, although you can drink plenty of water, black coffee, black tea, herbal teas and carbonated water. Diet drinks and sugar free gum are allowed but I wouldn't recommend them for the reasons I set out in a later chapter. Most people will find this one easier to do if the fast period runs through the night while they are sleeping, with a break of the fasting period being approximately six hours after you wake up. If you prefer to eat in the morning, of course, that is a completely viable choice with the Leangains program. This is fully adaptable to any type of lifestyle but it is important that you maintain a consistent window of time for feeding. If you don't, your hormone levels will be all over the place and you will struggle to stay with it.

What you eat and when you eat it during your feeding time will also depend very much on your workout times. On the days that you exercise, you should eat more carbohydrates than fat. On your rest days, it works the other way around. Keep your consumption of protein high on rest days although this will be entirely based on your gender, goals, age, activity levels, and your body fat percentage. Regardless of the specifics of the program you undertake, stick to whole foods for the biggest part of your calorie intake.

Pros

The biggest plus for many people is that, for the big part, the frequency of your meals really isn't important. In your feeding window, you can eat whenever you want. However, most people do find it easier to stick with three meals. It's what most of us are used to, and the eight to ten hour feeding window this program offers makes such a schedule very comfortable.

More than the convenience, this protocol stands out from the others in that is provides a higher level of hormonal management. How's that? Other intermittent fasting protocols like 24-hour or alternate day intermittent fasting are quite difficult to consistently adhere to on a daily basis but not the Leangains protocol. It's because the fasting time is much shorter at 14 to 16 hours only and not the whole 24 hours. This is especially fantastic for beginners and makes a great initial program (though it's been shown to be highly effective for even those quite well versed in intermittent fasting, so if you like it, by all means stick with it!). If you're able to sustain it longer compared to the 24-hour variants, you'll be able to increase your GH levels consistently and for longer periods. And that's what will help you improve your lean muscle mass to body fat ratio.

Another benefit of this protocol is consistency — you eat the same way each and every day. Consistency minimizes hunger volatility, i.e., hunger ups and downs, which lower your risk of quitting the protocol too soon. And speaking of hunger volatility, the reason why Leangains is able to stabilize it is because according to some studies, larger and infrequent meals tend to make people feel satiated for longer compared to the conventional smaller, more frequent meals.

Cons

There is a certain amount of flexibility in when you can eat but this protocol is quite specific on what you should eat, especially when you are working out. It can be somewhat difficult to schedule the strict nutritional plan and to schedule when you eat around your workouts and this can make things quite tough for some people.

Since the strength of this protocol lies in consistency, i.e., workouts are executed in a fasting state and the fast-breaking meal is always the post workout one — it goes without saying that one possible con is lack of flexibility. It can become rather impractical, to the point you may have to shift your open feeding window of opportunity to more inconvenient times of the day.

For example, say your first scheduled meal (breaking the fast) is at 7:00 a.m. If you only have an 8-hour window (10 for women), it means your last meal for the day should be at 5:00 p.m., which will give you 16 hours of fasting. There are some potential concerns for this set up. One is social. This schedule rules out practically all social dinners you may ever want to participate in. Can you imagine having dinner with your family or closest friends and tell them you can't eat? Good luck with that.

Another potential concern is that your feeding window is mostly within office hours. It'll be hard to eat most of your meals as such — unless you're practically doing nothing at work. And lastly, this may pose the challenge that the bulk of your fasting hours are right after your meals window has ended. You can potentially tweak the schedule, of course. Perhaps try breaking your fast at noon and packing a nutritious and filling lunch to take along, enabling you to enjoy eating until eight or ten p.m., depending on your gender. Leangains works well for beginners and for people with non-traditional schedules (students, night shift workers, etc.), but in the long term you might find the inflexibility too stifling and want to expand your horizons to include other options.

Eat Stop Eat

This method suits people whom already have a healthy diet but are looking for that extra boost.

How it Works

It all comes down to moderation. Yes, you can eat what you want but when you are offered a slice of birthday cake, stick to the one slice. There is no sense in eating the whole cake!

For this protocol, you will fast for a 24-hour period, on one or two days of the week. During this fast, you are to consume no food at all but you can drink as much as you want, provided the drinks are free of calories. Once your 24 hours is up, you can go back to your normal eating habits. Just carry on as you did before the fast, as if you hadn't just taken a day long break from eating. Timing is down to your personal preferences. Some people will find it easier to finish the fast at what is a normal mealtime for them. For others, it works just as well ending it in time for a mid-afternoon snack. Do whatever works for you and, if your schedule changes in any way, adjust your timings to suit the new one.

Fasting in this manner will cut your weekly intake of calories without having any real effect on what you can eat. The only effect is on how often you eat. It is important that, if you really want to succeed on this one, you do need to introduce regular workouts, especially some resistance training, even more so if you are looking to lose weight or change your body composition.

Pros

24 hours may seem like an awful long time to go without food but this protocol is actually quite flexible. To start with, you don't need to go at it all or nothing. For your first time, just go as long as you possibly can without eating and then increase this over time as your body begins to adjust. Start the fast when you are in a busy period and don't have time to stop and think about food. It becomes much easier and more natural feeling as time goes on and your body adjusts to the new habit.

Also, there aren't any foods that are not allowed. You don't need to count your calories and you don't need to weigh every piece of food that you eat. That makes this so much easier to follow because, you know that when the fast is over, you can eat normally again. That said, this is not an invitation to pig out and eat yourself stupid. This can be difficult to avoid if you had a problematic diet prior to beginning, as the combination of major dietary changes and total fasting for 24 hours can be very difficult to transition to. As such the Eat Stop Eat method works best for people who already have fairly healthy diets and enjoy maintaining that. Of course, it is quite alright to enjoy some treats or less than perfect foods now and again while on this plan, and because of that it is easy to follow, the risk of screwing up the fast is low and it tends to be very easy to incorporate into your lifestyle. I mean, how difficult is it to understand the only rule you'll have to understand, which is don't eat for 24 hours?

Another benefit of this protocol is caloric reduction. Consider if your daily caloric requirement is 2,500 calories, that's 17,500 calories weekly. So if you fast for, say a minimum of 2 days in a week, that's already a 5,000 calorie reduction for the week! Without much change in your lifestyle, you already lose close to 2 pounds a week. And supposing you were tempted to cheat by eating just a bit more than normal on your feeding days, the amount of calories you missed out on during the 2 fasting days is still more than enough to result in a significant caloric deficit for the week. Do it consistently week in and week out, month in and month out, it would be impossible not to see significant changes in your body's body fat levels. What more if you add an exercise program to it?

Oh, and more than just calorie management, this fasting protocol offers the benefit of improving insulin sensitivity and increasing growth hormones for body fat reduction and muscle mass gain. As mentioned earlier, the less frequently you eat, the lesser your body's need to produce insulin. When that happens often, you become more sensitive to insulin because there's little time for your body to be desensitized to it. And insulin sensitivity is key for losing stubborn body fat. This flies in the face of the popularly esteemed principle of eating frequent small meals daily.

Yet, you need more than just insulin sensitivity to really amp up your body's fat burning furnace. You also need growth hormones or GH, which your body consistently produces. But there are 3 specific times of the day when GH production is elevated: while or immediately after sleeping, after exercising for at least 10 minutes, and during or immediately following a fast.

What do these mean? This means if you secrete a lot of GH in your sleep and during fasting, then the obvious answer would be to continue your fast even after you wake up, extending your body's elevated secretion of GH. Couple it with exercise and get ready to enjoy significantly higher levels of GH — and fat loss or muscle gain.

Cons

For some people it will be very difficult to go a full 24 hours without consuming any calories. Some people find that they get extra cranky when they don't eat and they get some pretty annoying side effects as well — headaches, anxiety, fatigue — although these will go away as your body gets used to it. It is also more tempting to binge out when the fast is over and, although you can stop this. It takes an awful lot of self-control and willpower, something that not everyone has in abundance. If you decide to try out Eat Stop Eat, I recommend taking it slow at first. Limit yourself to just a couple of fast days a week to give your body (and mind) the time they need to adjust. For most people, the unpleasant side effects vanish within a few weeks and they start to enjoy all the time they save by not having to cook or eat on their fast days.

The Warrior Diet

This intermittent fasting protocol suits those people who like or need to follow a set of rules to be or feel successful.

The Warrior Diet (WD) was developed by Ori Hofmekler, which requires a 20-hour fast with a 4-hour feeding window. As you may have guessed by the name, it is supposedly inspired by the dietary habits of ancient warriors who interestingly enough weren't known to eat 5 to 6 smaller meals daily. According to Hofmekler, ancient warriors lived on only 2 meals at most, usually a large dinner and a small breakfast meal and it is this model that WD tries to emulate. Take note though that this assumption of ancient warriors' dietary habits is often criticized as being a counterfeit form of intermittent fasting. Why?

It's because of the relatively few hours in between the 2

meals — small breakfast and large dinner — of about 8 to 10 hours only, which most experts deem is too short to be considered fasting or enjoy the benefits thereof. For purposes of fat loss, this may work well, though, as it is likely to cut calories due to eliminating lunch and many types of snacks. But critics posit that if it's not long enough to be considered a fast, you may miss out on some of the other benefits exclusive to intermittent fasting.

Another reason why critics doubt the "fast"-ness of the fasting period is because it allows for small servings of protein, and raw fruits and veggies during the "fasting" window. As such, fasting purists and experts discount it as a legitimate intermittent fasting protocol. But if being shredded is all you're after, this is a good protocol to follow. Most people, however, choose to tweak this program to just have one big meal at night. This enables the plan to truly qualify as intermittent fasting and ensures that you can gain many of the benefits that a genuine fasting plan can provide.

How it Works

Expect to only have a feeding period of 4 hours per day, eating one large meal in the evening, and then to fast for the remaining 20 hours. However, although you only get one meal a day, you cannot eat exactly what you want because the type of food is also a key to the success of this method. The idea behind this is to feed the body with the required nutrients that it needs and that has to be done in sync with the circadian rhythms. The human species has been programmed to eat in the evenings, not during the day.

The 20-hour fast period is more about under eating rather than not eating so you can eat during this period. You can consume a couple of small portions of raw vegetables and fruits, drink fresh juices and eat some protein. The idea is to maximize the fight or flight response in the human body and this promotes a boost in energy levels, alertness, and stimulates the fat burning process. It effectively recreates many of the conditions that led to our ancient ancestors being so lean and fit and modifies it to suit a modern day lifestyle.

The feast phase of 4 hours is the overeating phase and is at night because it is designed to boost the ability of the parasympathetic nervous system to recuperate and rest your body, aiding digestion and promoting relaxation and calm. It also gives your body the chance to use the food nutrients to help repair your cells and boost the secretion of growth hormone. Our bodies naturally work on healing and rejuvenation of cells more strongly at night while we rest, and this plan utilizes the greater amounts of hormones released in the evening to ensure greater health.

Nighttime eating can also help the body to produce hormones and more efficiently burn off fat during the daytime fasting period. When you do eat, there is an order to the food groups that you eat. You should always start your feast with vegetables, fats, and proteins. Once you have consumed those three groups, if you do find that you are still hungry, then you can have some carbohydrates.

Pros

Many people tend to do this one because, although the fasting period is a long one every day, you can still eat some things, and this can make it a little easier to get through. The lower pressure combined with a more structured plan can make it an excellent choice for beginners to intermittent fasting. A high percentage of people who do this protocol have also reported a much higher level of energy and increased fat loss.

The Warrior Diet (WD) helps improve your sensitivity to insulin. As mentioned earlier, it's a very critical hormone for promoting muscle growth and fat loss. The more sensitive your body is to insulin, the higher your tolerance for carbohydrates and the better your body's nutrition partitioning (optimal calorie distribution between muscle and fat cells) become. It also improves your body's ability to use protein to build muscles, which ultimately leads to better fat burning. When your body becomes less sensitive to insulin, your risk for Type II diabetes and obesity significantly increases. Because WD effectively cycles short-term fasting and under-eating, your body becomes more sensitive to insulin. And the combination of WD with regular exercise during the fasting phase increases your body's sensitivity to insulin even more.

And speaking of burning fat, LSU researchers discovered the body's ability to oxidize, i.e., burn, fat improves when alternating days of normal calorie consumption and fasting, which may help burn 4% of your existing body fat in as little as 22 days. It also helps destroy the prevailing myth that eating late at night promotes fat accumulation and solidifies the belief that doing so can actually help you build more muscle than fat. This is because your GH production peaks at night while you sleep and when you eat before sleeping, you provide your body the necessary nutrients for maximizing the benefits of GH in while you sleep. Fasting throughout the day also helps increase your body's GH secretion.

The WD also helps you avoid excess energy build up. You don't have to count calories with the Warrior Diet and you simply trust your body to tell you when enough is enough. According to Hofmekler, your body actually thrives more on depleting its energy stores rather than on loading them. And for this reason, exercise is very beneficial for you while doing the Warrior Diet. Exercising depletes your body's energy stores and fosters an environment for your body to thrive. On the other hand, when you stuff yourself with so much carbs, you shut your stress response mechanism down. When this happens, you fail to immediately burn those calories and increase your risk for fat gain and inflammation, among other things. When you fast or under-eat throughout the day, you minimize your risk of building up excess energy by gradually depleting it the whole day.

While exercise is a very important aspect of burning fat and building muscle, nutritional stress is more important per Hofmekler. And by combining both, you enjoy their synergistic benefits and maximize your chances of successfully burning fat and building muscle.

Another benefit to this protocol is that like a 24-hour fast, fasting for 20 hours lets you enjoy the benefit of higher levels of growth hormones and generally lesser calories consumed, unless your intention is to bulk up. The warrior plan is better tailored to those looking to lose weight or to increase their endurance and fitness levels than those primarily trying to gain mass. Plus, given that you're probably going to eat just one large meal, the composition of such may not be as significant as long as you get the right amounts of protein. While you may eat less healthy food, you'd do well to minimize or avoid them altogether to maximize the benefits.

The Warrior Diet can also help you enjoy a longer life. According to the WD's chief proponent Hofmekler, nutritional stress like calorie restriction, under-eating or intermittent fasting can help lengthen the lifespan of just about any living organism from bacteria to the largest of animals. And this has something to do with what is referred to as mTOR or mammalian target of rapamycin, which is a type of protein that contributes to the regulation of cellular survival, proliferation, and growth. When you were young, mTOR helped you grow up into the mature (physically at least) adult that you are now. But as an adult, mTOR still plays a very important role in your risks for accelerated aging, cancer and diabetes. According to Hofmekler, mTOR can actually be detrimental to your health because it promotes unnecessary but adverse growth in your body that already matured and stopped growing. In other words, mTOR promotes unnecessary growth in a body that already ceased to grow.

According to studies, inhibiting mTOR can be significantly help reduce your risk for cancer. And guess what? Eating activates mTOR and food deficits inhibit it. Caloric restriction is — as of now — the only known intervention method that's believed to lengthen life in mice, flies, worms and yeast aging models. Further, mTOR inhibition can significantly contribute to the effective treatment of cancer and other cardiovascular sicknesses. For example, many cancer patients are prohibited from eating meat and dairy because it's believed that cancer cells get their nutrition from such foods. And alternating regular eating days and calorie-restriction ones — cycling between 56% and 144% of daily calorie requirements — extended the lifespan of people over 60 years old and helped strengthen their immune systems.

The last, and my most favorite benefit, is that it's pretty simple. I mean, how complicated can eating one big meal be, eh? The simpler it is, the fewer mistakes and the higher the chances of succeeding.

Cons

While it is nice to be able to eat a few bits during the fasting period, instead of going without altogether, the guidelines on what and when to eat can be tough for some people to follow in the long-term. The fact that it is quite a strict set of guidelines can also play havoc with your social life. Additionally, eating just one meal at night while following very strict rules on what you can eat and how to eat it, can be very tough, especially if you are one of those who doesn't like eating a large meal late in the day.

Another disadvantage to the Warrior Diet is though it's

simple, it's particularly hard to both fast throughout the day and stuff in all your day's worth of food in one large sitting — at least most of it. Think of going hungry all day and eating your breakfast, lunch, and dinner — total volume combined — in one sitting. Especially if you're coming from the 6-smaller-meals-a-day approach, this may seem overwhelming. One solution is to gradually transition into it by reducing the volume of food you eat during the day and reallocating the amount reduced to dinner until you have gradually and comfortably transitioned into the WD. Another solution is to eat more calorie dense foods, i.e., foods that pack more calories per unit of volume such as nuts and coconut oil.

Fat Loss Forever

This one is suited to gym lovers who also like a cheat day.

How it Works

If you are not happy with the intermittent fasting protocols we already talked about, then this one might suit you. It takes on the best parts of Leangains, The Warrior Diet and Eat Stop Eat, combining it all together in one eat method. get a cheat day every week, which is followed by a fast of 36 hours. Following that fast, the rest of the week is divided by each of the three protocols.

The suggestion is that you plan it so that your 36-hour fast coincides with a particularly busy period. This will let you focus on increasing productivity at work and not on the fact that you might be hungry if you don't eat for that long. You should also incorporate bodyweight training and free weight training to maximize your fat burning and muscle building potential.

Pros

Technically speaking, we all fast every single day, when we are not eating or we are asleep but most of us do so in a somewhat haphazard and non-consistent manner. That makes it very hard to gain all the rewards that proper intermittent fasting provides to us. This protocol offers up a weekly plan that incorporates several different methods, allowing your body to get used to a structure and to get the most out of the fasting periods. And, you get that full-on cheat day.

Cons

The cheat day must be followed in a healthy manner, i.e.

you do need to be able to eat only until you are moderately full, not completely stuffed to the gills with chocolate and cake. If you can't do this and you can't follow it up with a 36 hour fast, then this plan probably isn't right for you. On top of that, this is quite a specific protocol and the feeding window is going to shift every day, making it somewhat confusing to follow.

Alternate-Day Fasting or the Alternate-Day Diet

This is an easy way to fast, and it involves eating very little for one day and switching to normal eating the next day. A low-calorie day would mean a fifth of your normal calorie consumption. So, a fasting day will be about 400 to 500 calories for women and men respectively, because average calorie intake is about 2,000 to 2,500 calories. This can serve as a guide to calculate how many calories you should take on your low-calorie days.

To make these low-calorie days much easier to stick with, meal replacements are recommended because they are full of basic nutrients and can be easily sipped on for the entire day instead of eating groups of small meals. These meal replacements are to be taken for the first two weeks and after that, real food should be reintroduced on the low-calorie days. Then, as already stated, eat like normal the next day. As a precaution, avoid strenuous exercises during your low-calorie days. Stick to less rigorous workouts and save the hard work for your normal calorie days.

Pros

This fasting method totally guarantees weight loss, so you may want to try this if losing weight is your primary goal. Typically, people who reduce their calories by 35% can passively lose about 2.5lb every week.

Cons

Although it's quite easy to follow this fasting method, binging on normal-calorie days is quite common. To counteract over-eating, it's advised that you schedule your meals as much as possible so that you don't find yourself at a super-loaded buffet with an angry, grumbling belly.

The 5:2 Diet (Fast Diet)

The 5.2 diet entails eating as usual for five days and then limiting calories to about 500-600 for the remaining two days of the week. Also known as the Fast Diet, this diet recommends that men eat 600 calories while women consume 500 on fasting days. For instance, you can choose to eat regularly every day except Tuesdays and Fridays, where you eat only two small meals (300 calories per meal for men and 250 for women).

Pros

The Fast Diet is very flexible, and you are solely responsible for choosing your fasting days and how you prefer to share your calorie allowance on those days. Planning is also simplified as you can schedule your meals efficiently to ensure that you are consuming the right amount of calories. You could decide to do it as a main meal, or between breakfast, lunch and dinner. Since there are no banned foods, this means that the diet is not restrictive, and you can eat reasonably on non-fast days while eating very nutritious meals on fast days. This allows you to enjoy your favorite foods five days of the week and not feel deprivation. Also, because you don't have to be on a diet for more than two days, the 5:2 Diet is quite simple to stick to, knowing that you will eat normally within a day or two.

Cons

The low-calorie limit recommended for the fasting days does not give room for much food during the day, which means you may be foregoing some food groups in order to fit in with the stringent calorie schedule. Sometimes on non-fast days, some people tend to overeat to compensate for the limited food consumption on fasting days. Such overindulgence could render the fasting days pointless and could make it less sustainable in the long run. Another thing to note is that if your diet is already deficient, eating normally for five days may have no positive effect. To benefit maximally from the Fast Diet, you would need to improve on your eating habits overall. Additionally, the 5:2 Diet fails to address mindset or exercise which are critical components in the quest for sustainable long-term weight loss. As with other intermittent fasting protocols, the Fast Diet is not necessarily suitable for everyone, especially for pregnant women or people with insulin-dependent diabetes and eating disorders.

Spontaneous Meal Skipping

A less-structured intermittent fasting method is the spontaneous or convenient meal skipping. If the more coordinated fasting methods are a bit too daunting for you, you could start with this as a way to strengthen your resolve to fast. This mainly involves skipping meals every now and then, especially when you're not hungry or too busy to prepare a meal. Most people believe that if you don't eat very often (every few hours), your body will suddenly go into starvation mode and start to wither away. On the contrary, the human body is capable of surviving without food for extended periods, so skipping one or two meals from time to time isn't going to dramatically starve you. So if you wake up one morning, and you're not hungry skip breakfast and have a healthy lunch and dinner. If you need to go on a short trip, and there's nothing to eat, seize the opportunity and go on a short fast. Making this a habit is basically a more relaxed and spontaneous form of intermittent fasting. However, make it a point to eat nutritious and healthy foods when you do eat.

Pros

A recent study showed that eating normally one day, and reducing your calories on another day due to skipping meals can lead to a weight loss of about 8% of your body weight in two months. Skipping meals is a controlled eating plan that can be quite advantageous in that it reduces your calorie consumption without instigating a starvation response. Skipping lunch when you are at work, for instance, can be an excellent way to help you cope or deal with hunger pangs, which can never be avoided while dieting. Additionally, skipping meals as a form of intermittent fasting is not rigid in any way. If you get too hungry, an apple or orange can do the trick. Some people prefer not to miss lunch, but would rather reduce their calorie intake the next day which can also be very effective.

Cons

Some recent research has revealed that skipping meals during the day and eating a large meal for dinner is potentially unhealthy. The subjects of the study who were made to skip breakfast had a delayed insulin response and higher glucose levels when fasting.

There is quite a truckload of research that supports eating many small meals during the day to lose weight, instead of skipping meals. Evidence shows that eating often helps regulate your blood sugar levels, control your appetite and prevents you from snacking between meals.

Severe reduction in calories may cause the rate of metabolism to slow down. Few calories are required to maintain a healthy weight but make it harder to lose extra weight. This primarily explains the weight-loss plateau frequently experienced by dieters.

Skipping meals very often may lead to changes in behavior and moods. It's common to feel anxious, depressed, impatient, and irritable due to food deprivation.

Food for Thought

The human body needs time to adjust to a new schedule, some needing more time than others. When you first start, you should be somewhat cautious and start with a short fast, building it up gradually as your body gets used to it.

While these methods are very well known for incorporating specific feeding windows into your daily schedule, there are other ways to do the same thing but in a less rigid way. If you prefer to go with the flow of a day, follow the intuitive eating concept. Eat when you are hungry, not because you feel that it is necessary. Provided you are drinking plenty of water, your body will tell you when it needs food. However, do be conscious of still eating a healthy meal and of not overeating. You may be tempted to go for high calorie foods when you haven't eaten in a while and that will do you no good.

5 Top Tips to Starting Your First Fast

If you think that you want to give intermittent fasting a go, do keep these tips in mind when you do:

1. Stay hydrated. Make sure you drink plenty of water; not only will your body thank you for it, you will find the fasting periods much easier to go through.

2. Try to work your fasting period so it goes overnight. While it might sound like a lot to fast for 16 or 20 hours per day, it is easier when you consider that you will sleep for maybe eight of those hours.

3. Change the way you think. Instead of thinking that fasting is deprivation, think of it as giving yourself a break from eating for a while. That way you won't be focused on when you are going to eat next and what you will eat. Getting into this mindset will let you follow an intermittent fasting lifestyle long term

4. Overcommit yourself. This might seem a little odd but the best time to start a fast is during a busy period, not on a day off when you might be bored and tempted to pick at food. If you play your cards right, you can work out your schedule so that you are

so distracted you do not even think about the fact that you haven't eaten for hours. The first few times you do it are the hardest. By the time you are out of distractions and obligations, you will already be noticing and enjoying how healthy and energetic you feel while fasting.

5. Get to the gym. Intermittent fasting will work on its own but it will work even better if you work out a couple of times a week. You do not need to go overboard, just a simple workout two or three times a week will do the trick. Just make sure you incorporate bodyweight training in there somewhere.

How do you start?

There is a possibility that you could have done a lot of intermittent fasts in your life. Let us assume that you have consumed your dinner and slept right after. You woke up the following morning and have realized that you have overslept and rushed to work without consuming your breakfast. You have walked into the office and have been rushed into a meeting without being given a second to breathe. The only time you have a break is during lunch when you consume your first meal of the day. That pretty much counts as an intermittent fast since you have fasted for at least 16 hours already! So easy you likely barely notice when it occurs, which speaks volumes for the method of over committing to get started with fasting. There are quite a few people who do consume meals this way because they choose to live this type of lifestyle. They never seem to feel the pangs of hunger that most people do early in the morning.

Most people find it extremely simple to follow the 16/8 method which has been clearly explained to you in the seventh chapter. It is always good to start off with that initially since you will be able to sustain your health. The simplest approach of all is to fast whenever you want to. You could skip meals whenever you do not feel hungry or when you find yourself with absolutely no time to cook! You will not have to structure the fasting plan to obtain the benefits since you will be able to observe the benefits without a plan, too!

It is always good to use different approaches since you will be able to find something that you like most and will be able to stick to that very plan in the future. Have fun when you are fasting!

Chapter 8

The Food Basics of Intermittent Fasting

While you are beginning to embark on an intermittent fast, you will most definitely have questions with regards to what you can eat and when you can have your meals. First, let's talk about how much food is actually essential for living a healthy life.

How many meals a day is ideal for you? It depends on many factors, but generally speaking, with regards to the longevity of the lifespan, decreasing your risk for chronic diseases, and keeping yourself healthy for a long time, there is one sure short answer. Earlier conventional wisdom suggested that people need three square meals a day, with frequent snack breaks in between. However, there is scientific evidence to prove that this kind of continuous eating is the cause for rising obesity and diabetes. If you look back at our ancestors, they did not have access to food at all times, yet they were almost always healthy and robust. It does appear than intermittent fasting has a huge beneficial effect on your systems. Studies have been conducted with regards to eating multiple meals a day, which say that three meals might be too much for the body to deal with. People who skipped a meal, say breakfast or lunch, reported not much difference in their energy levels or their muscle mass. If anything, they felt lighter and more energetic throughout the day, and spent less time at the gym while observing similar gains.

Most practitioners of intermittent fasting advocate that you should miss one meal — either breakfast or lunch or dinner; any one meal, according to your preference and body systems. If you have a physically taxing job, you might want to eat a hearty breakfast and lunch and skip dinner. If you have a sedentary job, then your main meal might be dinner. But whatever you do, ensure that you stop eating two to three hours before your bedtime. Now, this method does not apply to growing teens and children, who need their full quota of food and nutrition. Unless they are overweight, in which case they might adopt a slightly watered down version of intermittent fasting. Make sure your kids eat wholesome food at meals, and cut down on sugary snacks and drinks as much as possible.

Why You Should Avoid Eating Late at Night

You keep hearing this — stop eating at least three hours before you hit the bed. There is some truth to this statement. For leading a healthy life, free of chronic and degenerative diseases, it's important that your last meal before bedtime is a good three hours before you actually sleep. Here's why:

In our body, mitochondria are responsible for burning the fuel which comes in the form of food. They convert the food into energy which is used by the body. These mitochondria create energy by generating electrons that are transferred to the ATP (adenosine triphosphate) molecules, the energy bed of the body. What happens is this — when you consume more calories than your body can use immediately, it results in the formation of extra free electrons, which slip back inside the mitochondria, as they are unused. Even so, they are extremely reactive and start killing off their host cells, the cell membranes and even cause DNA mutations. This, according to experts, is one of the causes of accelerated aging and a host of gastric related disorders.

To avoid this, keep your insulin resistance down by not eating three hours prior to your bedtime. While sleeping, your body uses the least amount of calories, so eating a large meal before bed will create an unnecessary burden on the system, which has to expend energy to digest all that food. If you have insulin resistance, then intermittent fasting is the best method to resolve it.

If you do not want to, do not skip dinner. If you are hard pressed for time and cannot manage the three hour rule, eat a light salad or fruit or simply have some milk before you sleep. Avoid sugary foods and other junk, though, especially right before bed. Keep your meal light on calories and high in nutrition, or switch to an early dinner if you find you really enjoy having evening meals.

Calorie Restriction and Your Health

Intermittent fasting is all about skipping a meal or rearranging your meal times, and this, according to research, helps you live longer. Studies have shown that calorie restriction over a longer period of time significantly changes the overall structure of your gut microbes, thus promoting longevity. This is also clearly correlated to a decrease in diseases, an increase in health improvements (including reduced inflammation, visceral fat, lower blood pressure, and increased immunity), and improvement of the quality of life.

How Intermittent Fasting Helps Your Body

Reduces inflammation, stress and cellular damage.	Improves the circulation of glucose pathways.	Reduces blood pressure.
Improves metabolism, efficiency, and	Keeps the LDL and cholesterol levels low.	Prevents or reverses the onset of type 2

significantly reduces body fat.		diabetes. If already present, it slows the progression.
Improves the immune system's responses and functions, and shifts the stem cells into a state of renewal.	Improves pancreatic functions.	Insulin and leptin levels and sensitivity are improved.
Provides benefits to the cardiovascular system akin to physical exercise.	Provides protection against cardiac diseases.	Keeps moderating visceral fat levels.

Gives a boost to mitochondrial energy pathways.	The ghrelin hormone, also known as the "hunger" hormone, is kept in check.	Helps eliminate sugar cravings and helps the body burn fat instead of sugar.
It promotes the production of the human growth hormone, which is also a fat burning hormone.	Promotes low triglyceride levels.	Boosts the production of brain derived neurotropic factor, which stimulates the release of new brain cells.

Intermittent Fasting Versus Calorie Restriction

Intermittent Fasting is not simply omitting calories from your diet. Intermittent fasting has added benefits. For instance, it is easier to follow than a diet. You eat wholesome and natural food, without sacrificing any food groups. When you restrict yourself from eating certain foods completely, you are going to be more likely to crave them, and you will have a very hard time sticking to your diet long term. When you consider calorie restriction, human beings have an innate resistance to weight loss, even when there is a severe calorie deficit. When the deficit ends, the body tends to over-compensate for the lean period and goes on a binge. The body has a tendency to go into "starvation mode" and the weight loss that should occur is resisted by the body. Intermittent fasting, when eased into properly, is a natural way to cut calories that does not result in your body trying to hang onto fat as it does when it thinks it may be starving. This is the reason why most diets fail (and often backfire) and intermittent fasting works.

Of course, it may seem rather contradictory. Calorie restriction promotes beneficial changes to the body, while on the other hand, chronic restriction may trigger our built in mechanisms to the extremes. What will work is a delicate balance between the deficit and surplus, while keeping in mind your body's systems and rhythm.

James-Sinclair

Chapter 9

What You Can and Can't Consume on an Intermittent Fast

There are some people that advocate eating proteins, fruits, and vegetables while on a fast but, technically speaking, you are not fasting if you are eating anything. Even having a cup of tea with honey in it could be classed as breaking the fast. However, just because you can't eat anything, it doesn't mean that you should avoid drinking. The most important thing to drink during a fast is water, at least eight glasses per day as a minimum. Not only does this keep you hydrated, it can also help you to feel fuller. Other drinks that don't contain any calories at all are:

- Black tea

- Black coffee

- Green tea

- Herbal teas

- Carbonated water

Do try to keep your caffeine intake down as low as you can, no more than two cups of coffee (around four cups of black tea and six of green tea) per day, too much is not good for you on an empty stomach and won't make you feel any better about not eating. Excessive caffeine, especially in the absence of food, can lead to an elevated heart rate, jitteriness, nervousness, and even paranoia, as well as other negative effects both physical and psychological. It's not worth it for the extra energy. It's a short-lived boost anyhow.

Watch out for the extra calories in milk and sugar. It might seem like a tough call to drink your morning coffee black but you will get used to it, especially when you start to see the benefits of your intermittent fasting regime kicking in. Adding a bit of cream here, a spot of sugar there, or even a bit of honey can have the effect of breaking the fast and sending your insulin levels back up. That means your body is not getting the full benefit of the fast. If you are doing a 24 hour fast, keep in mind that this is only for one or two days of the week so be strong about it and push on. You can do it if you really set your mind to it.

When you first start an intermittent fasting regime, you may suffer with headaches. This is not dehydration (unless you are not drinking sufficient water). Instead it is a symptom of withdrawal.

There is another good reason to watch your caffeine intake — caffeine is a diuretic and, unless you are regularly topping up with water, all those extra trips to the bathroom will take their toll. You may also suffer with a caffeine headache.

Avoid anything that is going to cause your insulin levels to spike. You know by now that insulin regulates how much fat is stored in your body so keeping it low while you do your fast ensures that your body is able to release the fat stores so they can be used instead of continuing to add to them. The places where this fat is deposited are in your stomach, bottom, thighs, arms and hips.

Some people advocate eating sugar free gum while on a fast and the idea behind that isn't all that stupid. After all, as a human race, we have been chewing leaves and gum tree sap for many thousands of years. However, on a fast, you should avoid all forms of chewing gum.

The regular type contains both sugar and calories, being sweetened, usually, with high fructose corn syrup. Corn syrup is a sugar form that you know better as glucose. Every time you eat a piece of this gum, it causes a spike in your blood sugar levels. The sugar free kind isn't much better because of the artificial sweeteners in it. A certain percentage of the population also has intolerance to something called phenylalanine, which is found in aspartame, and can cause a lot of health problems. Avoid it altogether.

The same goes for diet drinks, whether it's a can of diet soda or a cup of diet iced tea. Steer clear of it altogether while you are fasting. While a can of diet soda, or a stick of sugar free gum for that matter, doesn't have many calories, once again it comes down to the harmful chemicals that are in them and the negative effect they will have on your health. Diet soda has also been shown to actually raise insulin levels, which is the opposite of what you want.

Although one of the biggest benefits of fasting is the weight loss, it is also a good time to give your body a rest from the chemicals that are in so many of the foods that we eat on a daily basis. When it comes time to do a fast day, give the fake a rest and treat your body to a diet of fresh clean water, black coffee, and unsweetened teas.

At the end of the day, it is pretty simple to work out what you can and can't consume on a fasting day. If you have to ask yourself whether you can or can't have it, the answer is to steer clear of it. It's only for a set period of time, and the fast will give your body a necessary break.

James-Sinclair

Chapter 10

Health and Wellness Benefits of Intermittent Fasting

There are many benefits to intermittent fasting, not least the weight loss and muscle gain. However, there are also many other benefits that involve your health and wellness.

Simpler Life

If you're the hectic and busy type of person who's juggling a lot of things on your plate, intermittent fasting helps you enjoy better health and wellness without the burden of complicating your life even further with calorie counting and frequent eating. It can help you live a relatively simpler life by, among others, taking out one thing to think about after waking up — breakfast. You can simply down a glass or two of water and be on your way. This can free up time that you could use to squeeze in a morning workout, enjoy some quiet meditation or other spiritual time, or simply get to enjoy an extra hour or so of sleep before work, and who doesn't want that?

Even if you take on the protocol that simply makes you skip one meal throughout the day, it's still one less meal to worry about and hassle over preparations. One less meal's worth of shopping lists and money spent on ingredients. One less meal's worth of washing dishes. One less meal to plan, cook and stress about every day, which can be significant for most people. The time saved adds up more than you think — even if you only save an hour or so a day by skipping a single meal, when the year comes to a close, you will have an additional fifteen days' worth of hours that you previously spent doing nothing but eating.

Live Longer

It has long been believed that calorie restriction is a good way to increase a person's lifespan. This makes sense from a scientific and logical viewpoint because come to think of it, the human body was made to automatically seek ways to preserve itself. So when you purposefully subject your body to controlled hunger, you teach it to become more resilient in finding ways to live better and longer. And that's the beautiful paradox right there: starving yourself to live.

Again, intermittent fasting isn't to be confused with starving yourself to death by refusing to eat anything until you die. That's a fantastic way to substantially shorten your lifespan and you would be hard pressed to find any studies that advocate for such extreme "dieting." The kind of starvation we're talking about here is a temporary one that's controlled in such a way that you only subject yourself to just enough hunger as to be beneficial to your health — no more than that. The exact amount that is beneficial instead of detrimental varies from person to person. Know your body and do not push yourself farther than is safe or comfortable for you. Intermittent fasting merely facilitates the activation of many of your body's life extending mechanisms that are associated with calorie restriction.

Increase in Brain Function

Everybody can benefit from an increase in brain function and, conventionally, we have always been told that we should eat little and often to keep our brain completely focused and productive. We all know someone who eats to improve his or her creative thinking processes and to function more efficiently so you could be forgiven for thinking that intermittent fasting will do the complete opposite.

In fact, it will do the opposite of what you think it would do. In the same way that reducing oxidative stress in your body will help with aging, it will also help with improving your brain function. We mentioned the brain-derived neurotropic factor (BDNF) earlier; this is similar to a high quality fertilizer, except it's for the brain. It works by promoting neurogenesis, or the process by which neural cells are generated, and it increases your brain capacity. Normally, BDNF will increase with any physical activity that you do but intermittent fasting has exactly the same impact. It's simple, if you are not in a position to do a great deal of exercise, go on a fast.

Restriction of calories and fasting can stimulate new stem

cells and synaptic plasticity. The connections that are made between the neurons, through the synapses are made a lot more efficiently and a lot quicker. So, if you want your brain capacity increased, or you want to be able to make quicker connections or be more creative in your thinking, you should consider taking up intermittent fasting. Additionally, not stressing about food or planning your next meal in a few hours allows you to be more focused on your tasks at hand, boosting your creativity and your productivity.

Aging, Wellness and Disease Prevention

In the last few decades, diseases like diabetes, cancer, and others have come under a lot of discussion. They are some of the biggest killers in the world and we have seen an astronomic increase in the numbers of people who have these diseases. Medical practices the world over are in complete disarray and failing in terms of finances because so much money is having to be spent on caring for people and providing the right treatment for these diseases and their complications. It comes as something of a surprise to find that something as simple as intermittent fasting can have a profound effect on your risk factors in acquiring these diseases.

Diabetes

We did talk about this earlier and we know that one of the risk factors to diabetes is a high resistance to insulin. Because modern foods, frequently containing unexpectedly high amounts of added sugars, are so abundant these days, it is so easy to raise the blood sugar level beyond what your body can easily cope with and, to be honest, beyond what our ancestors would ever have achieved with their diets. As human beings, our bodies and hormonal systems were never designed to deal with a diet so high in added sugars. Because of this, our hormonal levels are totally unbalanced. One of the things that intermittent fasting does is re-balance those levels, thus lowering insulin resistance and lowering blood glucose levels. The reason this happens is (because we are eating less on an intermittent fast) we are not taking in so much of the deadly glucose and, over time, our bodies learn how to regulate our sugar intake, thus lowering our risk factor for type 2 diabetes. This can happen even when you eat as much as you want on a feast day or during your eating period — as long as you fast for between 16 and 20 hours, it will still work.

Heart Disease

Lifestyle is the biggest risk factor for heart disease, with poor diets and a lack of exercise. One of the biggest causes of heart disease is clogged arteries and a raise in LDL cholesterol. Research was carried out in Utah and it was found that people who fasted for a 24 hour period once a month were about 40% less likely to suffer with clogged arteries. That's a huge risk reduction for so little fasting. Imagine what will be accomplished with one day a week! Another study showed that, after just three weeks of following an intermittent fasting protocol, levels of HDL, the good kind, were raised in the study group and LDL levels were down. While a decrease in blood pressure has not yet been seen in human studies, it has been observed in a number of animal studies.

The Gender Gap

In all the studies that have been carried out, one thing has become apparent: women do not seem to respond to fasting in terms of insulin levels in the same way that men do, showing little or no improvement. Their LDL levels decreased in the same way though. This does not mean, in any way, that women should not do intermittent fasting; instead, it just means that either they won't see as much LDL benefit or they had a much better level of health before they started fasting.

The Hormones of Hunger and Intermittent Fasting

In order for you to have optimum health and well-being, you need a good balance of hormones and neurotransmitters and doing it the natural way is effective. That is what intermittent fasting does and that is how it helps you to curb your hunger and release the storage of body fat so that it can be burned off as energy.

Ghrelin

Most people have never heard of ghrelin but, when you start an intermittent fasting regimen, it is one of the single most important factors. Ghrelin is the hormone that makes you feel hungry and the body cells that are responsible for producing it work on a circadian rhythm. That rhythm is determined by your meal times so that means that you only feel hungry at times that you are used to eating, not necessarily because you genuinely are hungry. When you start a short-term fasting period, you will notice an increase in your metabolic rate. This goes back to our caveman days and is a response to make you get up and go look for food. It used to be necessary for survival, but these days most of us have an overabundance of food readily at hand. Intermittent fasting will train your body to release appropriate and optimal levels of ghrelin to support health and longevity, and lessen the urge tendency to eat just out of habit. Once your body is used to your fasting protocol, you will be able to optimize the levels of ghrelin that your cells produce and will find it much easier to eat less.

Leptin

Leptin is the joker in the pack — there's always one! Leptin is responsible for the thyroid hormones that work on regulating metabolism and fat loss. Leptin is actually produced in your fat stores and, as such, the less fat stores you have, the harder it is for your body to produce it. As a result, you may experience periods of stagnation, and reaching plateaus in body composition and physical fitness.

Leptin production can be prompted through intermittent fasting, during your feeding periods, and it can help you to burn off more body fat. From the perspective of body composition, it is better to eat a high level of carbs and calories on one day. Some programs advocate a "cheat day," during which you can eat what you like but you cannot overdo it. Yes, do have a cheat day but try not to stuff yourself silly with all the bad stuff (even though it may taste good!) For those of you that do high intensity training, incorporate your high calorie day with a day that you are working out.

Insulin

We know that insulin is important; too much of it puts you at risk of diabetes and we know that intermittent fasting can help to combat this. There are those that consider it best to eat carbohydrates in the early hours of the morning because of sensitivity to insulin. However, that is out of the window with intermittent fasting. Insulin sensitivity is much higher in the mornings because you have been fasting overnight while you sleep (unless you are one of those who sleep walks and eats without knowing it, of course!). Therefore, if you are doing a 16 hour fast, your insulin sensitivity will be much higher.

For muscle growth, it is best to eat carbohydrates late at night (just not within three hours of bedtime!) because an increase in carbohydrate intake at night will increase the amount of growth hormone that is secreted, thus helping with muscle repair.

Chapter 11

Things to Remember with Intermittent Fasting

To be honest, not too many people are willing to give intermittent fasting a try. It seems that the act of willfully and consciously depriving yourself of food is a really bad idea, especially when you feel hungry. We are heavily conditioned to feel that we should eat when we get hungry, especially if we want to build energy. We are constantly warned of diminished energy and unhealthy weight loss if we deprive ourselves of something so essential for life, and it can be very hard to break past these misconceptions. You know now that you only feel hungry because your body is conditioned to expect food at certain times and a regular intermittent fasting regime can knock this on the head. The first few weeks are going to be the most unpleasant for you so give these methods some attention as they may help you to overcome things and find intermittent fasting easier to do.

It's Mostly in The Mind

Intermittent fasting, as I said earlier, is very simple because you really don't need to count calories or prepare as many meals. In fact, you don't even have to eat upon waking up if you choose not to do so. At least that's how many people who are into it are doing it. But that's not to say it's easy...it is generally very hard. And most of the challenge comes from the mind. Part of the mental challenge is thinking:

·   How will I be able to function well at work or school the whole day if I don't eat enough or at all?

·   What if I feel lightheaded due to starvation and faint?

·   What if I get sick as a result?

Most people who have successfully incorporated intermittent fasting in their lives had similar thoughts at first, which they were able to eventually overcome when they realized that nothing happened even if they worried about it — that life went on as usual. That is not to say you will definitely not get any side effects — headaches and fatigue are particularly common, among others, but it's important to stick it out for a few weeks and to ease into it slowly at the start. If you give your body adequate time to adjust to your new lifestyle, you will likely not suffer any ill effects at all, and any that do exist are almost always mild and short-lived. No fainting or sickness as a result of fasting!

Mindsets are very powerful barriers, particularly beliefs like you need to eat frequently, that breakfast is the stuff that champions are made of and that going hungry is evil. These are messages drilled into us since we were small children, and they may very well hold true — for children, who are still growing and require more regularly-timed food. Sticking with the same fears your whole life, though? All of that is in the head — your head. Chances are, you just believe it and haven't really experienced the truth of those statements. I mean, you have very likely skipped breakfast a number of times before. Did you feel weak, sick or faint?

Did you even really miss it? Probably not. Test and challenge your preconceptions before you dismiss intermittent fasting. You may have been simply programmed mentally.

To successfully get ripped and enjoy greater health through intermittent fasting, it would be well to adhere to the advice given in the Bible: transform yourself by the renewing of your mind. When you believe differently, you act differently and start to get different results.

One Day at a Time

If you start off with the intention of doing intermittent fasting for the rest of your life, boy is it going to seem like too much. Instead, do this one day at a time. Anyone can get through one day of something unpleasant, so even if all your fears and uncertainties come to fruition, it's only for a day! It won't take you — and your body — long to find out that it isn't so bad, only being able to eat during a set window of time. Once you have done the first day, the next one will seem easier. And the one after that will be easier still. Before you know it, you will already be going full swing into an intermittent fasting regime without even noticing any difference.

Think Longer Term

Often times, we tend to look at the things we do on a short-term basis, i.e., hourly or daily. For successful intermittent fasting, it's best to plan on a weekly basis instead of daily or God forbid, hourly. An example is protein. When fasting intermittently, you don't have to worry about downing a protein shake within the golden 3-hour window of after working out, but within 24 hours, which makes it more practical and convenient.

One of the best things about intermittent fasting is that it totally debunks the myth perpetuated by most food and supplement manufacturers: that you need to eat every few hours for optimal health and fitness. Simply put, do you really think your body cares whether or not you eat every 3 hours or eat once or twice a day within a particular feeding window for as long as it gets the calories it needs? I thought so.

Thinking longer term — or slightly longer at least — helps you realize that you don't need to micromanage time-wise and that the difference between eating all throughout your waking hours and eating within a limited period of time every day isn't that significant over the long term. It also helps you achieve your desired ripped condition much faster, and, by cutting meals, you are buying yourself valuable time that you can use to train more or to enjoy more personal time.

Work Out Your Goals

Before you begin, determine your achievable goals. If you want to change your body composition, by increasing muscle mass and decreasing body fat, give the 16/8 method a go. Obviously, it's important to tweak your caloric intake and your training schedule based on your goals. Cut calories for weight loss, but be careful not to if you are trying to gain muscle mass. If you are looking at anti-aging and preventing of disease, do a 24 or 36 hour fast once a week. No matter what you do, do not fast for more than 72 hours.

Build Your New Regime Around Your Social Life

If you were to do your intermittent fast between 9:30 am and 5:30 pm, the normal working day, it wouldn't really work. For a start, you would be tempted to eat more and second, you would cheat more often. Consider your social life and make it easy on yourself — set your feeding period to something like 12 pm to 8 pm. You will find it much easier to stick to and, should you be at a meal with friends, it won't be an issue for you. Social pressures and temptations lead to the downfall of many good dietary plans. Intermittent fasting is definitely prone to failing due to your social life. Plan around it, and try to involve your friends and family and your new lifestyle and encourage them to support you. It will make a world of difference in sticking with your new habits over a lifetime.

Drink Water First Thing in the Morning

If a good deal of your fasting period is overnight, while you sleep, and it doesn't end until, say 2 pm the following afternoon, the best way to stop feeling hungry is to drink a big glass of water as soon as you wake up. Overnight, your body dehydrates and replenishing that water first thing will go a long way towards knocking hunger pangs on the head. Keep drinking it throughout the day, too, even once you break your fast at last. It will make you feel so much more energized and strongly diminish your desire to eat when it is not yet a feeding time.

Drink Tea and Coffee

When your fasting period encompasses a morning, drink some tea or coffee. Provided you are not adding any cream or sugar to it, you are not breaking your fast. This can feel more like an actual meal than simply water, which might help you stick with your goals, especially during your adjustment period. Drink it warm (or iced, if you prefer) and drink it black; this will help you to focus better and will get rid of those hunger pangs. Some people advocate starting the day with something like the Bulletproof® coffee, which contains MCT oil and butter. It is a very high calorie drink but the body can easily burn these calories off as energy and the coffee will not cause any disruption to your body's normal functions, like the repair of your cells.

Keep in Mind That You Won't Always Be Hungry

The hunger hormones are activated through habit more than genuine feeling of hunger. After about 4 weeks on an intermittent fasting regime, your body will get the message that you are not hungry when you are fasting and the hunger hormone secretion will slow down. Hunger pangs should actually begin to slow down in the first week and, from a psychological point of view, the thought that you will not always be hungry is a great start. So much of this is a simple placebo effect, so if you can convince yourself that you will be fine, you really will be fine.

Those who've embraced the intermittent fasting lifestyle have experienced that over time, their appetite and desire for food were reduced significantly, freeing them of any bad eating habits. They have experienced how it is to truly be in control over food and not being under its control. As such, they enjoy more freedom and flexibility now than when they were on a normal eating schedule.

Losing Weight Isn't So Hard

When you get used to eating less frequently, your body tends to generally eat less overall. The natural result is, unless you strategically want to bulk up, body fat loss and/or weight loss. Try as you might to attempt eating singularly bigger meals, you may be pleasantly surprised to find that it's becoming more and more of a challenge because your body and your mind would have been accustomed to generally consuming less food all day.

As such, intermittent fasting is both a very practical and

effective option for fat loss. It provides a very simple way of cutting down on total calories and without even having to change your general diet. Even if you get used to eating 1 or 2 bigger meals every day, those may not be enough to compensate for the loss of calories from the single meal you cut out. Essentially, cutting off one meal and eating a bit more on the remaining ones is often enough to create a significant caloric deficit for fat loss.

If you're the type who can't start the day without a glass of juice or cup of coffee, don't worry. You don't need to ditch it while fasting intermittently. Just make sure you stay under 50 calories throughout the day, which is the limit for being in a fasting state. The exact principle behind this number isn't clear but with enough reputable experts saying this is the case it is enough for me to roll with it. If you'll be having coffee or tea, stick to pure and unsweetened ones.

Train Less, Maximize Benefits

Often times, potency requires minimalism. Much like the strength of coffee or any alcoholic drink dissipates as you dilute it with water, the efficacy of your workouts during intermittent fasting may follow suit if you train too much. But how does overtraining look like in this context?

The obvious examples are exercising at very high intensity and for longer periods of time. When you exert too much effort (intensity) than what your body can currently handle under a fasting state, you run the risk of burning out, getting sick or being injured. Even at the right intensity, regularly working significantly longer than what your body can safely handle runs the same risk as excess intensity. Can you imagine if you do both at the same time?

What does the right intensity look like? Generally speaking, you'd feel very uncomfortable — lightheaded, very tired and weak or prolonged muscle soreness — during or after working out if you over train. A relatively objective way of determining if you're exercising at moderate intensity, which is ideal, is through the talk test. If you can still carry a normal conversation while working out albeit with some difficulty, that's moderate. If you're able to carry a conversation in the same manner as you would over coffee with a friend or if you can barely say a word while catching your breath, then you're under (low intensity) or over (high intensity) training, respectively.

A good way to focus your training is to prioritize compound exercises, i.e., those that involve the most number of major muscle groups to execute the movements. Examples of these would be burpees, which recruit most of your major muscle groups.

Another way of prioritizing your exercise is to go for those that utilize the biggest muscle groups, particularly legs and back. Why? The bigger the muscles, the more calories are required to contract them. That's why doing 1,000 crunches aren't enough to get you ripped, but running daily for at least 30 minutes, which involves the biggest muscle group, the legs, can help you do so. Keep in mind that you cannot truly target specific areas as much as is sometimes implied by supposed experts. If you are working out and lifting regularly, you will see gains in all your muscles, not just the ones you are targeting the most. As such, it makes sense to grant priority to the larger muscle groups to enjoy the maximum gain.

Choose an Indulgent Day

Some people like to have a cheat day and eat whatever they want. While you should do this sensibly, you can have days where you eat more carbohydrates and calories — just choose the cleaner food sources, like sweet potatoes, almond butter, and dark chocolate. Don't feel bad if you want a break to enjoy some foods you cut out now and again — depriving yourself completely is a good way to kill your motivation and stop fasting altogether. An occasional treat, provided you have designated times and days for it to not interfere with your plan, will not jeopardize your fitness goals.

Keep Busy During a Fast Period

This is one of the biggest reasons why it is easier to have your fasting period run overnight, because you are sleeping and not thinking about eating. If you are awake, keep busy, occupy yourself with something. This does get easier over time, of course, as your body adjusts to simply eating less you will find that your thoughts turn to food less frequently than before. That said, when you first start this regime, you are not going to help yourself if all you are thinking about is the fact that you can't eat for so many hours!

Fast(ing) Productivity

Don't be surprised to find that your most productive times

of the day are within your fasting period. As most people expect mental performance to take a dive during the fasting periods, this will probably be one of the most pleasant surprises you will experience while fasting intermittently.

It seems that reduced body burden (less digestion, more energy for other things including thinking) helps in improving mental clarity while under a fasted state. This is consistent with reports of many people who fast for religious purposes — that they feel more connected to their deity and are able to think better and clearer. Regardless of the reason, I believe you can expect your personal productivity to exponentially increase while fasting intermittently.

It Matters What You Eat

While intermittent fasting is an excellent way to improve on your health, it really won't matter a jot if you don't eat sensibly and properly in your feeding periods. Try not to eat too many carbohydrates and eat plenty of protein and good fat, along with fresh vegetables and fruit. When you do eat carbs, focus on whole grain, healthy options with no added sugars. Avoid overly fried or greasy foods and ensure you are getting balanced nutrients (take vitamins or supplements if needed, or alter your diet).

Intermittent Fasting is NOT for Everyone

So don't believe that it is. See how you get on, how it goes for a week or two first and then decide if it is something that you can do. Don't feel like a failure if it isn't and if you simply can't go on with it. Listen to your own body and figure out what you feel healthiest and most energetic doing. Intermittent fasting is a fantastic lifestyle choice for many people, but there are many other solid healthy options you could select instead. If you are one of the few people who does not come to like intermittent fasting, for either physical, emotional, or mental reasons, take a break. Give it a fair chance and if it's not working for you, move on to something that does work for you and your lifestyle.

James-Sinclair

Chapter 12

Ready to Start?

Not so fast! Before you get all excited about the benefits of intermittent fasting and dive straight into it, I would strongly recommend that you take a couple of weeks to get your body acclimatized to what you are about to do to it. It is common when you first start, to feel very hungry at times and, as such, it is best if you work into it by gradually cutting your feeding window down over a couple of weeks. If you go from a feeding window of 14 hours straight down to eight, it is not going to be very pleasant.

For the first week, cut a couple of hours of that window; perhaps wait an extra two hours in the morning before you have breakfast. Better yet, try to have a light dinner a few hours earlier than normal if you can find the time. This eliminates nighttime eating and extends your fast time at the same time. That's something you should be able to do. Your hunger pangs, if you get any at all, will only be mild ones and you can knock those on the head with a cup of black tea or coffee or a big glass of water.

When it comes to eating, stick with what you normally eat or, if you can, gradually eliminate some foods from your diet and substitute them with others.

On week two, cut another two hours off your feeding window in the mornings so, instead of eating at 6 am, you will now be waiting until 10 am for example. Just think of it as brunch rather than breakfast and keep on drinking that water. You can also mix the two. Have breakfast two hours later and dinner two hours earlier. To easily extend your fast time.

The third week is the last part of the acclimatization and this is where your feeding window will be down to eight hours. By the end of this third week, you will know if intermittent fasting is right for you and you will be able to make your plans accordingly.

FAQS on Intermittent Fasting

These are some answers to the most common questions about intermittent fasting.

Is This a Faddy Kind of Detox Type Diet for Quick Weight Loss?

No, it is not. Obviously, you will lose weight on this because you are consuming less calories but it will be more of a gradual and steady loss. Your body will undergo some kind of a detox because you are giving it a break from chemicals and you will be eating better foods. Intermittent fasting is more of a lifestyle choice than a diet.

Am I Allowed To Drink Liquids While Fasting?

Of course! Water, tea, and coffee can be taken during the fasting period. Also, non-caloric beverages are good. You may add little amount of cream or milk to your coffee and tea but refrain from adding any sugar. Coffee is highly recommended during a fast because it can minimize hunger pangs.

How Many Calories Should I Consume?

The simple answer is: less than you do normally. You do

not need to worry too much about calorie counting but do make sure you keep it in check. Eat real foods instead of processed ones and you will automatically be on your wat to becoming a winner. Eating fewer meals means eating fewer calories anyway and, provided you don't go stupid and pig out on your feeding periods, you will still experience a deficit in calories each week.

Is Intermittent Fasting Based On One of Those Low Carb Diets, Or Any Other Diet?

Not particularly, no. Fasting is simply eating and how you eat during your feeding window is up to you. If you want to go low carb then go ahead. Most people tend to find that eating whole foods gives the best results but anything is possible with intermittent fasting. It's all about training your body to no longer require food 24/7.

Am I Allowed To Take Supplements During A Fast?

Sure. Remember though, that some supplements are more effective only when taken with meals. So you may need to learn about the supplement's requirements before taking them.

Is It Safe To Exercise While Fasting?

Yes. You can work out while fasting. Branched-chain Amino Acids (BCAAs) are recommended before a fasted workout.

Can Fasting Cause Muscle Loss?

Muscle loss is typical for all weight loss methods which is why keeping protein intake high before lifting weights is necessary. A recent study revealed that intermittent fasting results in less muscle loss than a regular low-calorie diet.

What Exercise Should I Be Doing On an Intermittent Fasting Regime?

The best kind is intensity training where you use a short burst of high energy and effort. Continue with your normal exercise and fitness regime but build in a few high intensity exercises as well. This will boost your body's response for burning fat and growing muscle mass, as well as encouraging a much better use of glycogen and amino acids. However, do not go overboard with the exercise, particularly cardio exercise as you can easily burn out. Additionally, be sure not to neglect strength training. If you're looking to put on muscle mass a combination of intense weight training and intermittent fasting will have you looking ripped in no time. Short high intensity workouts a couple of times a week will work wonders.

Will Fasting Decrease My Metabolic Rate?

No. Short-term fasts have been shown to increase metabolism. However, fasting for extended periods may repress metabolism.

Can Children And Teenagers Fast?

That may not be such a good idea. Children are still growing, physically and mentally, and fasting may harm these natural cycles. It is best to consult with your child's pediatrician if weight is an issue.

I Can't Go Without Breakfast!

You don't need to go without breakfast; all you do is move the time that you eat it, that's all. And, if you eat a large meal the night before, you might just be surprised at the level of energy you have when you wake up. The biggest concern that people have about intermittent fasting is that they have had it ground into them that you must not miss breakfast, you must eat a large breakfast and you must eat every few hours. There is no science to support any of this.

So, Why Do I Keep Hearing That You Should Eat Every Few Hours?

When you eat, your body will burn off a certain amount of calories so it was thought that, by eating more often, you were burning off more calories and, as a result, would lose more weight. There's a bit of a problem with this though, and I'm sure you can see it already.

You see, the calories that you burn off when you eat are in direct proportion to how much you eat and how much food your body is having to process. So, if you eat six small meals that total 2,000 calories, your body burns off the same amount of calories as it would if you ate 2 large meals that totaled 2,000 calories. It does not matter whether your calories come in the form of six meals or one; the result will be the same.

If I Don't Eat for 24 Hours, I'll Die!

This is nothing more than a mental barrier and it is the biggest thing that stops people from trying intermittent fasting. First off, fasting is actually a religious practice and has been done for centuries. Medical practitioners have been saying for thousands of years that fasting is beneficial to the body. It isn't a new fad, and it isn't a market ploy to get you to spend vast amounts of money on something that doesn't work (in fact, it may very well wind up costing you less than a conventional diet and food choices do). It does work and it has been around for years.

Secondly, the reason why fasting might seem an odd thing is because not many people talk about it. That's because there's no money to be made in telling you to cut down how much you are eating. The most promoted diets are usually the ones that tout eating nothing but their meals, their shakes, their herbal remedies. With intermittent fasting, you do not have to buy any of that since you will be eating the same foods you ate before. You don't need to buy supplements or special diet foods and, as such, it really isn't something that is marketable.

Third, if the truth is known, you've already fasted without even realizing it. Apart from the fact that you fast when you sleep, how many times have you slept in on the weekend and eaten later than normal? Some people practice this every weekend. You eat your dinner on a Friday night and then don't have anything else until lunchtime the next day. You fasted for 16 hours and you didn't even realize. Did you suffer any ill effects from those late mornings? Unlikely.

Finally, even if you don't intend to take up intermittent fasting, I would suggest that you do one 24-hour fast. Just one. It's enough to teach you that you will survive just fine if you don't eat for a day and it may just convince you to give intermittent fasting another go.

I Work Shifts, Can I Still Do Intermittent Fasting?

Technically, yes but if your feeding period is going to keep changing, it won't do your metabolism any good. Try to make it so that you eat at roughly the same time every day, that's the best you can do with shift-work. If possible pack healthy snacks or lunches and eat them at work when you are there during feeding periods. With careful planning you can still keep things fairly consistent with a difficult schedule.

Do I Need to Count Micros While on an Intermittent fast?

Not but do keep in mind that, just because you can only eat during a set period of time, that is not a free for all. If you continue to eat more calories that you are burning off, you will gain weight.

What If Something Happens and I Miss My Feeding Window? Do I Need to Change My Window the Next Day?

There will be times when it is unavoidable so that you can't stick to your window because things happen. All you do is eat when possible and then go back to your normal time the following day. Try to be consistent but don't feel like a failure if life gets in the way. These things happen sometimes and as long as it is atypical it will not undermine the benefits of fasting.

What Effect Will Intermittent Fasting Have On My Workouts?

You don't need to change the way you exercise just because you are on an intermittent fasting regime. Some protocols require you to train in specific ways but, if the plan you choose to follow doesn't, just carry on as normal.

If I Don't Eat Frequently, How Will I Survive?

You will surely survive even if you don't eat for a whole day. This particular mindset is the biggest drawback for most people which can hold someone back from giving intermittent fasting a shot, even though it's not that difficult. Fasting has been practiced for centuries and boasts of numerous health benefits. You can stay without food for a day or two, and life will go on as usual.

Will I Lose My Strength?

Absolutely no, in fact, many people who go to the gym have reported that they actually have better performance and strength levels! If you combine strength training with intermittent fasting, relying on principles like avoiding nighttime eating and timing your workouts around your fasts for optimal gain, you will likely find that your strength increases once you start fasting. Yet another way that intermittent fasting benefits you.

I Feel So Ill — What Can I Do?

The whole idea of intermittent fasting is that your diet should be much easier, certainly not harder. If you feel that bad, then stop doing it, it's that simple. As I said before it isn't for everyone and it might not be for you. Try to give it a chance before you quit. Some side effects are common while your body adjusts, especially if you started fasting cold turkey. But if negative health impacts persist, do what's right for you and for your health.

I'm a lunch lover. I can never skip it. So, how do I try this method?

If you don't want to, do not skip lunch. Just change the time of when you eat your lunch foods. For instance, if you regularly have your lunch at one pm, push it back to three or four, and later to a late evening time. Pick a time which suits you. Plus, having a big dinner the night before proves surprisingly effective in giving you energy. Finally, you can still love lunch at any time. Enjoy your favorite lunchtime foods, but just enjoy them at dinnertime. That sandwich will taste just as good when it isn't sunny out anymore!

Do I need to do anything differently as a woman?

Not really. Although, it's usually said that a wider eating window is more favorable for women during daily intermittent fasting. A woman may get better results by fasting for 14 hours and eating for 10 hours while a man my fast for 16 hours and eat for 8. Still, whether you're a woman or a man, you're advised to experiment and find what works best for you. Follow the signals that your body gives you.

But how can I NOT eat for 24 hours and still live?

The most obvious problem is the mental barrier people have, which prevents them from fasting. It is not as difficult as it sounds. Here's why: fasting has been around for centuries now, and science has proven the health benefits for fasting for periodic intervals. Many religious people throughout time engage in fasting regularly, sometimes even to rather extreme degrees in comparison to the plans we've discussed here. Very few of them have ever died from it, and most of them emerge from their fasting times feeling refreshed and closer to their respective deity. It's not something new and is certainly not a fad which has recently cropped up. The reason why people don't talk much about it is because, well, frankly, who wants to tell people NOT to eat? With supplements, exotic foods, and processed goods rampant in our culture today, it is simply not marketable to tell people to stop eating for a while. And surprisingly, you might have fasted without your knowing it. What about all the times you slept in late or had a late brunch or had a late dinner and skipped breakfast the next morning? We don't even think about such things. We sometimes eat lunch later than usual, and don't realize it. That's a 16 hour fast and we don't even think about it.

To get started, try the 24 hour fast first. Teach yourself that it's okay to skip a meal sometimes.

Chapter 13

The tips and tricks you will need!

You have been given tons of information on intermittent fasting and you have probably started screaming inside your head! You may be worried about how you will be able to cope up with the diet you are going to start now. Well, stop worrying! This chapter gives you all the tips and tricks you will need to ensure that the fast works for you instead of going down the drain.

Stop Freaking Out!

You will have to get rid of your thoughts about the number of hours you can fast. Stop asking yourself if you should only fast for 9 hours instead of ten hours! Stop worrying about how consuming a single French fry during your fasting period is going to affect it. Please relax! You have an extremely smart body that will adapt itself to any changes you may make to your lifestyle.

If you are looking at consuming lunch or breakfast one day and want to skip it the next, go ahead! If you are aiming to become an athlete or aiming towards becoming very strong and muscular, you will need to be very rigid with respect to your diet. If you are looking to lose some weight, add some muscle tone, or extend your life and better your health, fasting is a lot more flexible and easier than you fear. You should just chill!

Do not worry about people staring.

You may have just begun the fast and would have found people staring weirdly at you. You will probably go out for lunch with a couple of friends and hey, you have stopped eating lunch. Now what do you tell your friends? They will definitely ask you tons of questions; they are your friends after all! You will probably have to take a lot of time to explain yourself, but if they do not understand what you are saying, then embrace the weirdness! Even if they have trouble accepting or understanding it, they will get used to it over time. Social lives and friendships are rarely destroyed due to intermittent fasting, so relax and just laugh off any jokes about your new lifestyle.

Keep yourself busy.

If you have just started your intermittent diet, you will probably have trouble trying to curb your thoughts about hunger. You may sit around and begin to wonder about how hungry you are and will probably crave some form of food. So, let me give you a certain pattern that you could use during the first few days of your fast!

1. Right before the first few hours of your fast, you should consume a huge meal! An extremely huge meal let us call it a monster meal. You will stop worrying about when you are going to eat next!

2. You could try sleeping a decent amount of time since you cannot worry about hunger when you are dreaming! Maybe start on a weekend and enjoy a lovely Saturday morning sleep in and fasting.

3. Try to keep yourself busy during the day to avoid worrying about your hunger.

4. Last, but not least, keep telling yourself that you do not need to think about hunger since you are a strong person! Remind yourself of the reasons you are doing this and remember that you are fully capable of accomplishing those goals.

You can consume beverages with no calories.

Yes, you have been asked to fast. But, this does not mean that you cannot drink water! All you have been told is to avoid consuming any food with calories in it! You could drink green tea in the morning and even during your fasting period if you want to. You could also drink black tea or coffee during your fasting period. Always keep it simple!

Always listen to your body

Each person has a different response to intermittent fasting. You will never be able to gauge how your body will react to the fasting by comparing yourself with people around you. You will need to see how your body is reacting and make the changes required.

1. Are you concerned about having lost too much muscle mass? For this you will need to start keeping a track of your strength by undertaking strength training routines to assess the intensity of your strength.

2. You could buy fat calipers which would help you track how well the fat has started to burn away in your body!

3. Always keep a track of your calorific intake! You will be able to see how your body has started to change with respect to the quantity of food you eat. Additionally, by counting your calories you can ensure that you really are cutting calories when you fast and not just making up for the missed meals by overeating.

Do not expect to see miracles!

This is a mistake that every beginner makes when he or she starts any fast. You will want to see results in a week or two. But, what they forget is that a fast is not the only thing that will help. You will need to understand the fact that there are many other factors which will affect the way you lose weight or even the amount of weight you will lose. You have to look at intermittent fasting along with other healthy habits, like exercise and sleep, which will ensure that you lose weight consistently. Even if you are working out, sticking to your fasts, and doing everything right, it still takes time to see real, noticeable results. Give it at least a month and ideally longer before you decide you are not losing enough weight from fasting.

Motivate yourself

You have been told above that you should not expect miracles. Well, this may seem easy but you will start feeling terrible when you find no changes after a week or two. This is when you will need to motivate yourself and tell yourself that you are doing a great job. You have to keep forging ahead and will need to give yourself the strength to stick to the diet. You could always have a buddy with you who will help you — perhaps a coworker, family member or friend you can get on board to join you in fasting, or at least to encourage you and urge you to stick with it when the going gets tough. That said, if such a person does not exist, then you will just need to push yourself forward!

James-Sinclair

Conclusion

So, there you have it — intermittent fasting in a nutshell. Despite what you may think about not eating for so many hours, it will not kill you and, trust me, you will not feel all that hungry either. The real trick is to make sure that you eat properly and eat the right foods during your feeding window and, that you drink plenty of fluids, especially water.

Intermittent fasting has so many benefits and very few, if any downsides. A lot of people have gotten fantastic results with some of the intermittent fasting methods listed in this book. Still, it really will not work for everyone so do not feel put out if it doesn't work for you. It may be that you are on the wrong protocol so try another one. If you are fasting for 24 hours twice a week, give the 16/8 a go and fast for 16 hours every day. Even just twelve to fourteen hours or so of fasting can be beneficial — skip breakfast, or dinner, if you cannot bring yourself to skip both or find that doing so does not work for you personally. It is easier if you make sure that your fasting period covers your sleeping time. If you work nights, change your feeding period to the nighttime and your fasting period to the day, when you are sleeping. Also, do not forget that the effect of intermittent fasting will be rendered pointless if you binge on junk food during eating periods. Whether fasting or not, the quality of your food is absolutely essential.

One thing I must stress is this — do consult with a physician before you start any intermittent fasting protocol. Intermittent fasting is completely safe for the vast majority of people, but there are some factors that could encourage your physician to recommend against it. Certain medical conditions and certain medications prohibit fasting and you may end up feeling worse or your medications may not work for you. Additionally, if you are very thin, especially if that is due to an eating disorder or if you are prone to weakness and fainting, you may need to gain some weight or otherwise ensure your previous conditions are deemed medically safe before you begin. Even when you consult a physician while on the diet, you may find that there are no changes that have been made to your body. Our bodies all change at different rates. Some of us can lose weight easily and some of us struggle more than others to gain muscle mass. You might find one of your desired results not appearing as quickly as you thought (and hoped) that it would when you began your fast. It is during this time that you keep yourself motivated since quitting the diet will never help you in any way! Good luck!

James-Sinclair